THE
ANTI-CANCER
DIET

THE
ANTI-CANCER
DIET

Donald R. Germann, M.D.
with Margaret Danbrot

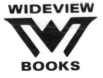

WIDEVIEW
BOOKS

First Wyden Books edition: September 1977

First Wideview Books edition: January 1980

Library of Congress Cataloging in Publication Data

Germann, Donald R.
    The anti-cancer diet.
    Bibliography: p.
    Includes index.
    1. Cancer—Prevention. 2. Cancer—Nutritional
    aspects. 3. Nutritionally induced diseases.
I. Danbrot, Margaret, II. Title
RC268.G35   616.9'94'05   77-22254
ISBN 0-87223-545-9

CONTENTS

Introduction: You Can Reduce Your Cancer Risk

What if I told you that diet is linked to more than one-half of all cancers in women and to at least a third of all cancers in men? What if I went on to say that 239,000 new cases of cancer each year, in the United States alone, might be avoided if only the victims knew how to choose their food more wisely? What if I ended by saying that you yourself could reduce your chances of developing the disease by 80 percent if you made some simple changes in your own diet?

I think you'd sit up and take notice. I think you'd want to know how I had arrived at those figures, and then you'd want more specific information about the dietary changes involved. Most of all, you'd want to know how you could incorporate some of those changes into your life.

Well, that is precisely the kind of information you will find in this book. As you read on, I know you will be heartened by a growing sense of optimism about your prospects for living a long, healthy, cancer-free life—just as I was when the weight of accumulating evidence first made me aware of the tremendous role diet can play in the prevention of this mysterious disease.

You see, many of the most important findings of recent cancer research lead us to conclusions that are good news indeed!

Though we still can't offer cures for many cases of the disease, and though for many types the exact cause is not yet clearly understood, we now believe we have a powerful weapon for *protecting* ourselves against it. It's a weapon that is available to each and every one of us, without a prescription and at no extra cost to our pocketbooks, our time or our energy. Just as important, it's one that is 100 percent safe in terms of our health. That new weapon is the food we eat, or in some instances, the food we avoid.

I want to emphasize that I'm not alone in this view. When I say that with proper diet 239,000 new cases of cancer each year might be prevented, I'm not simply giving my own personal estimate. Far from it. Those figures and the conviction that the food we eat is perhaps the single most important factor in the development as well as the prevention of cancer represent a consensus of belief held by many of the most highly qualified and respected people in the fields of public health, preventive medicine and cancer research. In fact, in July of 1976, officials from the National Cancer Institute, the American Health Foundation, Harvard University, the Massachusetts Institute of Technology and the Wistar Institute of Philadelphia testified to that belief before the United States Senate Select Committee Hearings on Nutrition and Human Needs.

Those experts, let me hasten to add, were not recommending the widespread consumption of any new "miracle" foods. If they were, you'd have known all about it, for the press would have picked it up in a flash and the day after the hearings we'd have seen banner headlines from coast to coast announcing the news that "FOOD X PREVENTS CANCER." Nor was that group of distinguished scientists testifying *against* any particular food. That, too, would have made headlines.

In fact, the cancer specialists who met in Washington to speak before members of the Senate Select Committee didn't even have a lot to say about food additives, except to note that when used at present levels their potential for causing cancer in human beings has been grossly exaggerated. Now that *should* have made the front pages. A lot of people are worried, very worried, about the chemicals in their food and would have been grateful for any reassurance about food additives and contaminants. But no. Most of the men and women who decide what's news and what isn't chose to soft-pedal that particular piece of information. (Just as they made a big deal over the 2 percent increase in the United States cancer rate in 1975 but have all but ignored the 5 percent decrease during the first six months of 1976.)

What those cancer specialists *did* tell the senators was that the "standard American diet"—not any one food, mind you, but our affluent diet itself, high in fat, protein and highly refined carbohydrates and low in roughage—is possibly a causative factor, and certainly a predisposing factor, in literally hundreds of thousands of cancer cases each year, and that if we ate differently, we'd see a change in our cancer mortality rate. It should have been shouted from the rooftops. But it wasn't.

That lack of attention is just one reason for my decision to go ahead and write this book. Not that there's a dearth of information for the lay person about cancer. There's plenty of it. Unfortunately it tends to be scattered and inconsistent. Hardly a week goes by without another story about some new chemical in our environment that may cause cancer. Though I intend to remain a harsh critic of environmental chemicals and to insist as loudly as anyone that harmful chemicals be banned, I'm more concerned about the fact that other equally important information—no, far *more* important in terms of the lives that might be saved because of it—simply isn't getting through. What amounts to a major cancer breakthrough has come to pass. But everyone is looking in the other direction.

True, that breakthrough has to do with prevention, and prevention is never as dramatic or exciting as cure. But until we have more cures, we need to do everything possible in the way of prevention. I know. As a radiologist, much of my work has to do with the diagnosis and treatment of cancer. Time and again my colleagues and I are forced to confront the unhappy fact that to be a five-year survivor of this disease is to be in the minority. As things stand now, no method of treatment is as good as not having cancer to begin with.

In this book you will find suggestions for a better way of eating that can substantially reduce your own and your family's risk of developing cancer. Taken together, these suggestions constitute the Anti-Cancer Diet. It is based on research that indicates beyond reasonable doubt that certain kinds of food make people more vulnerable to the disease while other foods seem to protect against it.

Among my major sources of information are a collection of papers read at the Symposium on Nutrition and Cancer* at Key Biscayne, Florida, in May, 1975; material presented at an international conference on the detection and prevention of cancer, held in New York in April, 1976; transcripts of the United States Senate Hearings on Nutrition and Human Needs, which took place in July, 1976; reports read at another Symposium on Nutrition and Cancer† in New York, in November, 1976. (Readings from these conferences and hearings are readily available to professional and nonprofessional alike.) In addition to these major sources, I've made use of information gleaned through a thorough search of recent medical literature.

Of course, important work in the field is still going on. The last word on the relationship between diet and cancer isn't in yet, and it may be years before our understanding of it is complete. For that reason, I've no doubt that some few members of my profession will feel that it's too soon for the Anti-Cancer Diet, that we shouldn't suggest making dietary changes until we've arrived at some more precise explanation of *why* the food we eat is such an important factor in the development of some forms of the disease.

I also know that there will be many, many others who will agree with me that to sit on this potentially lifesaving information—to keep it from the public until certain theories have been perfected—would be irresponsible. I believe we cannot afford to wait—just as we counseled people to stop smoking before every last shred of evidence on the major cause of lung cancer was before us. In making a few modest changes in the way we eat, we have absolutely nothing to lose and a high probability of gain.

We know enough now, right this minute, to start making certain recommendations. Many of us—doctors, scientists, researchers and others with access to the new findings—have already begun to modify our diets along Anti-Cancer lines. I'm hoping that a careful reading of this book will convince you and your family to do the same.

Donald R. Germann, M.D.

* Sponsored by the American Cancer Society and National Cancer Institute.
† Sponsored by Columbia University.

The Anti-Cancer Diet at a Glance

VEGETABLES—As much as you like. Choose as often as possible (preferably twice daily) from the cruciferous vegetables—cabbage, cauliflower, broccoli, spinach and turnips, among others —as well as celery and dill. These are the vegetables that reduce the incidence of tumor formation in laboratory animals and may have a similar effect in human beings. Vegetables provide the greatest amount of bulk when eaten raw and unpeeled.

FRUITS—Again, as much as you like. Fresh uncooked fruits are preferable. Apples, pears, peaches, apricots, plums and the like should be eaten with the peel.

CEREAL GRAINS—In general, eat more of the unrefined whole grain products. These include whole grain breakfast cereals such as oatmeal, all bran and shredded wheat, as well as whole wheat bread, brown rice, and bran to sprinkle on top of or mix in with pancake batter, muffins, meat loaf, soup, et cetera.

LEGUMES—Peas, beans (including soybeans) and peanuts can be used often. Their calorie content is moderate, their vitamin and mineral content is good, and they're excellent sources of vegetable protein. Dishes in which a legume is combined with a cereal grain provide high-quality complete protein and are a nice change of pace from animal protein.

RED MEAT—No more than six four-ounce servings per week of lean beef, pork, lamb or veal.

POULTRY—One or more four-ounce servings per week of chicken or turkey, skin removed. Ideally, chicken or turkey would be used to replace red meat for several meals during the week.

FISH—Two or more four-ounce servings of nonoily white-fleshed fish per week. Ideally, fish should be used to replace red meat at several meals.

PROCESSED MEATS—Ham, bacon, frankfurters, corned beef and many lunch meats not only have a high fat content but also contain nitrates and nitrites. Therefore, they have *no place* in the Anti-Cancer Diet. On those infrequent occasions when eating them is unavoidable, make sure to include a food high in vitamin C with the meal.

ORGAN MEATS—Liver, sweetbreads, kidneys, and brains are good sources of many vitamins and minerals but of all foods they're highest in cholesterol. Avoid them completely.

MILK—For adults, no more than two cups of *skimmed* milk per day.

CHEESE—To be used with discretion as a meat substitute. Skim milk cheeses are always preferable to whole milk varieties.

FATS AND OILS—Use as little as possible. When a fat or oil is necessary in cooking, choose corn oil margarine or liquid vegetable oil.

NUTS—High in vegetable protein and a good source of many vitamins and minerals, but unfortunately also too high in fat to be used in large amounts.

COFFEE—No more than five cups per day; coffee should be drunk before or between meals rather than as an accompaniment to the food.

TEA—No restriction, but never to be drunk scalding hot.

ALCOHOLIC BEVERAGES—No more than four one-ounce cocktails or mixed drinks per day (at an ounce of liquor per drink), or half a bottle of wine, or three cans of beer.

SOFT DRINKS—One or two bottles of dietetic (sugar-free) soda per day is fine. Regular soda (with sugar) should be avoided by people who must watch their weight, are diabetic or have elevated triglyceride levels.

CAKES, COOKIES, PASTRIES AND OTHER FOOD MADE WITH HIGHLY REFINED FLOUR AND SUGAR—To be avoided for several reasons. Their calorie content is high while they offer little in the way of nutritional value. (They're deficient in most vitamins and minerals, protein, fiber.) They also often contain large amounts of fat or oil. Angelfood cake is the exception. Choose fresh fruit, dried fruit, sherbet or gelatin desserts.

PART

I

EATING THE ANTI-CANCER WAY

1

The Truth about Chemical Food
Additives and Contaminants

Way back when word first got around that I was working on a book about food and cancer, various people—friends, neighbors, a few of my colleagues—just assumed that it would be another outraged diatribe against the use of chemical additives. When I told them that, no, I was planning to write a very different kind of book, that in fact one of the major points I wanted to make was that food additives and contaminants contribute very little, if anything at all, to the cancer problem in this country, they were taken aback.

"But don't you read what it says in the newspapers?" they'd protest. "Isn't it true that the cancer rate has gone up since food additives came into widespread use? Don't some of those chemicals cause cancer in animals?" And so on. And on. One person even went so far as to hint (in a jocular, tongue-in-cheek way, to be sure) that this project might have been initiated and partially subsidized by one of the big chemical companies.

That's not the case, of course. I have no interest at all in influencing public opinion in ways that would take some of the pressure off the manufacturers of chemicals used to process and preserve our food. On the contrary, I am very pleased that after so many years of not caring, so many people are now concerned about what goes into the food supply.

But I do worry that for some consumers healthy concern has become a kind of paranoia. Living in fear of what *they* (the food processors and manufacturers and, by default, the federal government) might be doing to us is bad enough. Worse is the possibility that that paranoia might get in the way of our coming to grips with the *real* problem—which is not the additives but the food itself.

It's about time, I think, that we try to put the issue of additives and contaminants into more realistic perspective.

First of all, what are they? In general, a food additive is a substance or combination of substances intentionally included in food in order to improve it in some way. Contaminants are substances that accidentally come into contact with the food. There's a distinction between the two. Yet with all the recent speculation about the possibly harmful effects of certain chemical additives, some people have a tendency to lump them together. In their minds any packaged or processed food listing a chemical as one of its ingredients has been "contaminated."

Part of the confusion arises from the word *chemical*. It has a decidedly negative connotation these days. But chemicals per se aren't bad. Food itself is chemicals. So are our very own bodies. Just as some chemicals or combinations of chemicals can do us harm, others are beneficial.

For example, some very recent cancer work indicates that a few chemical food additives may be *anti*-carcinogenic, that is, actually work against the onset of the disease. The story never got into any of my hometown newspapers, so I'll assume it's news to you, too. But first, a little background information.

Years of experimentation with laboratory animals have yielded some valuable "givens." Researchers know, for example, that when certain carcinogenic (cancer-producing) chemicals are administered to certain test animals, a certain type of cancer will develop in a certain percentage of those animals.

Working with some of this information, researchers have found that several chemical compounds of what we call the "antioxidant" type appear to *suppress* the cancer-causing effects of a variety of potent chemical carcinogens. The most extensive work of this kind has been done with a group of compounds called "phenolic antioxidants." Butylated hydroxyanisole and butylated hydroxytoluene—BHA and BHT for short—are two extremely common food additives that belong to this family of chemicals.

In one kind of test researchers administered a known carcinogen directly to the target tissue of an animal. (This is done by injecting the carcinogen into an organ or painting it onto the skin or, where the target tissue is the stomach or intestinal tract, feeding it to the animal.) The cancer that would ordinarily have developed as a result of exposure to the carcinogen was suppressed in those animals whose diets included five parts per thousand of BHA or BHT.

Similar results were obtained in other kinds of tests, using carcinogens that tend to cause cancer at sites far removed from where they are administered. (Good examples are the carcinogens that are given orally but which result in tumors of, say, the mammary glands.) Again, five parts per thousand of BHA or BHT in the animals' diet tended to suppress the development of cancer.

To be sure, these tests are done with laboratory animals under strictly controlled laboratory conditions. As we all know, what's true of animals in a lab isn't necessarily true of human beings in real-life situations. No scientist ever claims to have found a cure or preventative for anything solely on the basis of studies done with mice or rabbits. Animal testing only provides something to go on, clues that may point in the right direction (but also often lead up a blind alley).

BHA and BHT and their role as cancer suppressants need to be investigated more fully. So for the moment at least, I'm not going to recommend that you gulp down enormous quantities of food containing these additives. The fact is, even if you did you couldn't get into your daily diet the five-parts-per-thousand dose that suppresses cancer in animals. Still, I see no reason to go out of one's way to avoid them.

Another aspect of the BHA-BHT story should be mentioned here: the two compounds have been known to cause allergic reactions in some people. Because of this, many of the more outspoken consumer advocates favor banning them. However, BHA and BHT allergies are about as common as allergies to milk or rice. In other words, they're very rare. It's *possible* that at some time you or a member of your family might experience the discom-

fort of an allergic reaction to these additives, but it is highly unlikely.

Let's not forget that allergic reactions to eggs, shellfish, strawberries and wheat are fairly common and that many babies are
allergic to cow's milk. While we can sympathize with anyone
whose diet is limited by allergies, the fact that some people react
badly to a particular food doesn't warrant taking action that would
prevent others from eating it. (Of course, anyone who has already
experienced an allergic reaction to BHA or BHT should carefully
read the list of ingredients printed on the package or label of every
processed food item and avoid anything containing these additives.)

As of now, it looks as though BHA and BHT have a lot more
going for them than against them. They do the job they are meant
to do—which is to stabilize fats and thus retard spoilage. They are
safe for most of us. (Though undoubtedly troublesome to those
who suffer from them, the number of BHA and BHT allergies is
statistically insignificant.) And the possibility that they may have a
role in suppressing cancer in human beings is exciting, to say the
least.

What about the more than eight thousand other chemicals listed
as food additives in the *CRC Handbook* (the "Bible" of the
additive industry)? Which ones are good? Which ones are bad?
And how do we make any sense out of the conflicting opinions
about them? Unfortunately, in the case of many additives, the
answers are not nearly as clear-cut as they are for BHA and BHT.
But we don't need to consider them all, chemical by chemical, to
gauge the strength of their threat to us as cancer-causing agents.

In general, we can say that a good food additive is harmless and
necessary and a bad one is harmful and/or unnecessary—which
doesn't tell us anything we don't already know. The uproar over
food additives arises out of trying to define what we mean by
"necessary" and "harmless."

The purist would say that *no* food additive is necessary and cite
the fact that human beings endured for thousands and thousands
of years without adding chemicals to what they ate. (It's the same
line of reasoning that prompts remarks such as "If people were
meant to fly, God would have given us wings.")

The purists have a point. If each family grew, hunted and

cooked its entire food supply from scratch, additives would indeed be unnecessary. But given the way things are, there's a very real need to retard spoilage of food that is processed at one time and place and eaten somewhere else weeks or months later. We also need other additives to replace nutrients that may be lost during processing. Less necessary, but considered desirable by some, are the additives that improve the flavor, appearance and texture of the food.

A 1958 change in the food and drug laws came as a kind of official recognition on the part of the federal government that the use of chemicals *is* necessary and unavoidable for the provision of an adequate food supply. It permits the use of chemicals that improve our food and food technology—provided those chemicals are safe at the level of intended use. It stipulates that new additives must be proven safe before being offered for sale and makes clear that the manufacturer, not the federal government, must foot the bill for safety research. The amendment also provided for the development of the GRAS list. GRAS is an acronym for Generally Recognized As Safe. Any substance on the list is considered to be just that. The GRAS list was put together by scientists and is constantly being reviewed.

At about that same time the food additive amendment was passed the "zero tolerance" concept was established for potentially dangerous chemicals: any chemical that produces tumors in laboratory animals at *any* dose level must be considered unsafe. By the late fifties scientists had already identified many of the potent carcinogens—the ones that consistently and under many different test conditions produce tumors in animals. Now they were to go after the weak or low-level carcinogens.

A weak carcinogen is a substance that causes a relatively low incidence of tumors in the animals tested. (In other words, where a potent carcinogen might produce fifty tumors in one hundred test animals, a weak carcinogen might result in only one or even fewer.) In addition, with a low-level carcinogen massive doses and very long periods of exposure are usually required to produce cancer. This is where it gets confusing.

Many weak carcinogens cause tumors in some kinds of test animals but not in others. Often the sex and age of the animal is a critical factor. For instance, a certain chemical might produce tumors only in infant female rats, while male rats, older female rats and all others species of test animals appear to be unaffected by it. To further complicate things, some weak carcinogens produce tumors only when they are administered in a particular way—perhaps when they are injected under the animal's skin—but not in other ways, such as when they are fed to the animal.

We still have no good way of determining whether a substance that is weakly carcinogenic for one kind of animal will be more, less or not at all carcinogenic to people. Neither can we predict with any degree of accuracy whether it follows that a substance that produces tumors when painted on the skin of an animal will likewise produce tumors when fed to the animal—or when eaten by human beings. If there is a pattern, it has so far escaped us. It's this lack of precise knowledge that turns the question of whether to ban or not to ban a particular chemical into a pitched battle that rages on for months or years.

To get an idea of how complicated the issues are, let's imagine a hypothetical situation. Suppose that large amounts of a certain chemical painted on the skin of rabbits produces a low incidence of cancer in young male rabbits only, while other rabbits and all other test animals are unaffected by it. Should we prohibit the use of very small amounts of that substance in our food?

If the substance is not of any great importance to begin with, the answer, I think, has to be yes. Some of the dyes that are currently under investigation come to mind here. Surely we can all easily adjust to less colorful food.

But what if we're talking about a substance like saccharin? For many years now saccharin has been a great aid to diabetics and people watching their weight. There is no evidence whatsoever that saccharin (or any artificial sweetener for that matter, cyclamates included) has ever caused cancer in human beings. We have known for some time that when saccharin is fed to rats for two generations an increase in bladder cancer can show up in the second generation. When saccharin makes up 5 percent of these rats' diet, bladder tumors occur in 14 percent of the test animals (normal incidence is about 3 percent). And in March 1977 saccharin was banned by the FDA. They had no choice because the 1958 Delaney Amendment clause to the Federal Food, Drug and Cosmetics Act requires that:

No additive shall be deemed to be safe if it is found to induce cancer when ingested by man or animal or if it is found after tests which are appropriate for evaluation of the safety of food additives to induce cancer in man or animal. . . .

"Appropriate tests" are not defined and it is implied that "tolerance" should be zero.

This is one of many examples of the ridiculous nature of the zero tolerance rule. People would have to consume 800 12-ounce bottles of diet soda per day to get the dose of saccharin comparable to that given rats. I feel saccharin is important to the health and well-being of the public. Without it, our annual sugar consumption, which is already too high, will increase.

The question of what to ban should be based on the balance of benefits versus risks, not on a preconceived irrational dictum— even if such a dictum is easy to administer.

The question of whether to ban or not to ban is sometimes answered in ways that seem downright bizarre. Consider the chemical diethylstilbestrol, DES. A few years ago it was discovered that many young women whose mothers had received rather large doses of DES during their pregnancies developed cancer of the vagina. As a result, the FDA imposed controls on the then common use of DES by ranchers to promote the growth of cattle. In a recent article in *Preventive Medicine,* Dr. Thomas Jukes discusses the rationality, or irrationality, of the FDA decision. Small doses of DES do not produce vaginal tumors. In order to get enough DES from beef to produce tumors, we would have to eat our total body weight in beef liver weekly. Yet at just about the time the FDA decided to control the use of DES in cattle, the "morning after" pill was approved. Trace amounts of the chemical found in beef liver are minuscule compared to the amount of DES in the pill. Despite this apparent inconsistency we must understand the FDA has one set of rules for food and another for drugs. This is rational for we purchase food on faith and drugs for a special reason. These separate rules make it possible for the FDA to ban saccharin as food but permit its sale as a drug. Unfortunately, we need saccharin in food processing. Its availability over-the-counter as a drug is better than its total loss but as such its use will be awkward and more limited than desirable.

When a carcinogen is fed to test animals, it tends to produce *liver tumors*. This is no accident. In all animals, human beings included, the liver functions as a kind of purification plant, filtering out unfriendly bacteria and viruses and detoxifying poisonous substances. In a sense, the liver is the body's first line of defense. As such, it's the first organ to be affected by carcinogens in the food supply.

What are we to make, then, of the fact that cancer of the liver is quite rare in the United States and other western countries where chemical additives are in widespread use? Can additives be ruled out as a significant causative factor in the liver cancer we do have?

The most common kind of liver cancer in the United States, hepatoma, is found either in infants or in people who have suffered from cirrhosis of the liver for long periods of time. Angiosarcoma, another kind of liver cancer, is extremely rare. In the seven years from 1966 to 1973, there were only seventy-four cases reported in the United States and two of them were linked to vinyl chloride. (In fact, it was these two cases and an intense study of the industry that resulted in controls on the use of that chemical.) Approximately thirty more such cases have been found since 1973. The cancer that arises in the biliary ducts within the liver tends to be secondary to biliary tract disease—which means that the cancer usually develops after and as a result of some other liver or biliary disease.

The point is that if food additives are a major cause of cancer, it is not cancer of the liver, the one organ we would expect to be most vulnerable to carcinogens in our food.

Another way to evaluate food additives as cancer-causing agents is to compare the cancer rates of countries where additives are used liberally with the cancer rates of countries where additives are strictly controlled.

We can do this by taking a look at the situation in the Scandinavian countries. Denmark is one of the most conservative nations in the world in the use of food additives. Danish government regulations prohibit the addition of anything but salt to cheese, stipulate that only sodium benzoate may be added to egg products and are equally strict about other chemicals in food. Far more liberal are neighboring Norway and Sweden. In fact, their food laws are much less restrictive than our own. Apparently Norwegian and Swedish manufacturers, processors and importers are limited more by their own consciences than by their governments' regulatory agencies.

The three countries—Denmark, Norway and Sweden—are geographically and ethnically similar. From this we could expect that their cancer death rates would be roughly comparable. But the statistics tell another story.

Norway, with its liberal food laws, has 235.98 cancer deaths per 100,000 people in the population per year. Sweden, with food laws similar to those in Norway, has 243.70 cancer deaths per 100,000 per year. Denmark, with its strict prohibitions against food additives has a cancer death rate of 297.29 per 100,000 per year—a figure that is almost 20 percent higher than its two relatively unrestricted neighbors.

If additives were a major factor in causing cancer, we would certainly see less, not more, cancer in Denmark. At the very least it seems that the Danes have not been especially rewarded for their efforts to keep additives out of their food.

As for chemical pesticides and fertilizers, our most notorious sources of food contamination, large numbers of them have been introduced into the environment during the last thirty years or so. Some of them are "degradable," which means that with time they lose their chemical identities and revert to simpler, more innocuous compounds. Others we call "stable"; they remain in the environment unchanged for long periods of time and may be passed from the soil to water to air to animal. Both kinds tend to enter into human biology, either as residue on fruits and vegetables or in our drinking water. Some are thought to be carcinogenic.

Highly suspect almost from the time they were put on the market is a group of pesticides of the chlorinated hydrocarbon type, including aldrin, dieldrin, chlordane, heptachlor and DDT. They were intended to improve agricultural productivity, but many were also used in the home to get rid of unwelcome insect visitors. All are chemically stable. Once disseminated, they tend to collect unchanged wherever they happen to land. Worse, they accumulate in the fatty tissues of all types of animals, including human beings.

That some of these chemicals are carcinogenic to test animals is beyond argument. Dieldrin causes tumors in animals when given at one tenth part per million, the lowest level yet tested. (Apparently there is no such thing as a safe dose level of dieldrin—at least not for laboratory animals. Mice developed liver tumors after having been fed small doses of it for only two months.) Other tests indicate that aldrin and dieldrin are carcinogenic to rats as well. Aldrin, dieldrin, heptachlor and chlordane were taken off the market in 1970.

DDT is a little different from the others in the group. Like them, it's a stable compound that builds up in the tissues of animals and people. But whether DDT is carcinogenic is still at issue. It has been estimated that in providing the means for controlling the Anopheles mosquito, which spreads malaria, DDT has saved more lives than any wonder drug yet invented. Thus, it's easy to understand why the withdrawal of this pesticide from the market was an unwelcome event in many areas of the world. Already in some localities malaria has once again become a major health problem. For people who must weigh the risk of malaria today against the possibility of malignancy in twenty or more years, the reluctance to give up DDT is understandable. The fact that there has been no evidence whatsoever indicating that DDT has caused cancer in human beings only complicates the situation.

The truth is, there has been no evidence that any chemical insecticide or fertilizer causes cancer in human beings. I mention this, not because I think it was a mistake to prohibit the use of some of these chemicals (in matters of health I am about as much in favor of playing it safe as anyone can be), but because the information may be reassuring to people who are troubled by the thought that cancer is mainly the result of food contamination over which they have no control.

Graphs 1 and 2 should be reassuring as well. I've included them to give you a better understanding of cancer rates in the United States and how they've changed over the past thirty-five years or so. Chart A indicates the incidence of various kinds of malignancy for men, Chart B for women.

First of all, note that lung cancer is on the rise for both men and women. For men the incidence of this kind of cancer began to increase in the late 1930s—about twenty years after World War I, when great numbers of American men first began to smoke. For women the incidence of lung cancer began to increase in the early

1. Age-Adjusted Cancer Death Rates *
for Selected Sites, Females, United States

1930-1974

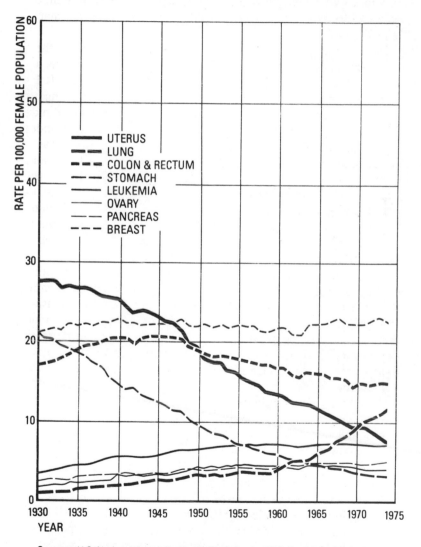

Legend:
- **UTERUS**
- **LUNG**
- **COLON & RECTUM**
- **STOMACH**
- LEUKEMIA
- OVARY
- PANCREAS
- BREAST

Y-axis: RATE PER 100,000 FEMALE POPULATION (0–60)
X-axis: YEAR (1930–1975)

Sources: U.S. National Center for Health Statistics and U.S. Bureau of the Census.
*Standardized on the age distribution of the 1940 U.S. Census Population.
Reproduced by permission of American Cancer Society, Inc.

2. Age-Adjusted Cancer Death Rates*
for Selected Sites, Males, United States

1930-1974

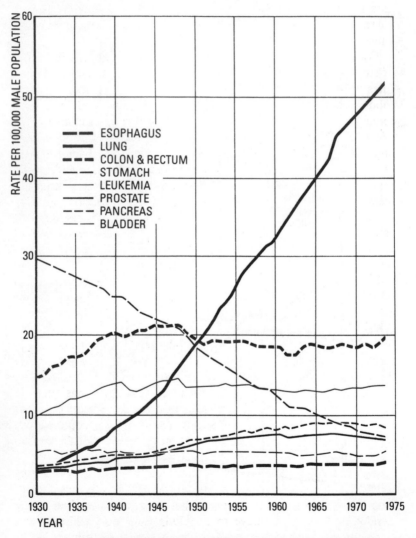

Sources: U.S. National Center for Health Statistics and U.S. Bureau of the Census.
*Standardized on the age distribution of the 1940 U.S. Census Population.
Reproduced by permission of American Cancer Society, Inc.

1960s. It's increasing even more rapidly now. Again, we have a twenty-year lag, this time between the 1940s, when smoking became socially acceptable for women, and the time when the unhappy consequences began to show up.

In the case of cigarette smoking and lung cancer, the charts give us a striking illustration of what happens when a new carcinogen enters our environment. We get an equally dramatic picture of how cancer rates fall when carcinogens are withdrawn.

For example, note that for both men and women, the incidence of stomach cancer has decreased for the last few years. The falling rates are thought to be due to a number of factors, most of them food-related. For one thing, nitrite levels in our food have been reduced. (We'll be taking a closer look at nitrites in chapter 16.) We've also had great improvements in methods of food storage and preservation, which have resulted in reduced bacterial contamination. (No, we don't believe that bacteria cause cancer, only that certain bacterial conditions set the stage for it.) Your refrigerator may be an important cancer prevention tool.

The charts show a small increase in a few cancers, namely, cancer of the prostate, pancreas and ovary. There are theoretical explanations even for these moderate changes, and we will go into them in subsequent chapters.

Finally, note that the incidence of all other kinds of cancer has stayed pretty much the same over the last thirty-five years. To me and to many others this lack of fluctuation is extremely important. We've seen how the incidence of cancer went up in a matter of twenty years or so after the introduction of a potent carcinogen (cigarettes) into our lives. It's been well over twenty years since the use of modern food additives and agricultural pesticides and fertilizers became widespread, and as of now there has been no corresponding change in cancer rates that would indicate that they have caused cancer in human beings. (Some of the contaminants that occur in nature—not man-made—have very important human cancer implications. They will be discussed later.)

Needless to say, I hope that we can identify new cancer-causing substances long before we see any telltale rise in the incidence of the disease. I'm honestly optimistic that we can do just that. At the same time I think we have to conclude that food additives and contaminants are not a major—or even a significant minor—cause of cancer in the United States. You and I are not victims of big food interests or federal government laxity, as writers of scare books and articles would have us believe. We are not helpless. We have the means of protecting ourselves from cancer within our grasp. It only involves changing some of our eating habits.

Ironically, I think some people will resist these glad tidings. If we could continue to blame the cancer problem on food additives and contaminants, we could do one of two things: demand the banning of more and more of them, or sit back and with a sigh of resignation hope we'll be among the lucky ones. Either is easier than making a commitment to changing the way we live. By the time you finish this book I hope you will be convinced that that commitment is worth it.

2

The Food-Cancer Connection

In the skeptical seventies I can't expect you to take up the Anti-Cancer Diet on faith, just because I say it's better for you. The idea of eating to prevent cancer may be a new one to you. Certainly it's a novel concept in traditional conservative medical circles. For a long time reputable members of the medical profession believed that the kind of food we ate—provided we got enough of the vital nutrients—had little to do with whether we stayed healthy or not. Only food faddists, quacks and others outside the mainstream of medical thought suggested otherwise.

So why are we having second thoughts about the connection between diet and disease? What's happened to change the minds of some of our best experts about the role of nutrition in the development of cancer? Why are so many of them now convinced that our eating habits are among the most important factors—if not *the* most important factor—in determining who will succumb to the disease and who won't?

The answer involves the research of dozens and dozens of dedicated and talented men and women working in many branches of medical science. To recount the whole story in detail from beginning to end would take several books of this size, filled with complicated charts, graphs and equations that many of you wouldn't want to wade through. Therefore, I'm going to simplify and present only some of the most important theories and evidence. (If you are of a mind to take a look at some of the scientific source material, by all means use the Bibliography at the back of this book as an aid in locating it.)

Cancer is presumed to be a disease of modern civilization. Statistically, this is difficult to prove, since very few records were kept prior to 1900. However, when we look at the few surviving primitive societies and compare their cancer rates with ours, the difference is readily apparent. Their cancer mortality rates are much lower than ours. Some of the difference is explained by the fact that people in the modern, affluent societies tend to live longer. (Cancer occurs most frequently in older people.) Still, even when mortality rates are adjusted to take age into account, we find that the more affluent and complex the social order, the higher the cancer rate.

Enter the specialists in the medical discipline called "epidemiology." Epidemiologists study diseases as they occur in particular localities. They're the experts who seek to discover how flu spreads from city to city, why heart disease is so much more common in some countries than in others and what circumstances lay behind the fact that only guests and employees at a certain Philadelphia hotel were stricken with last summer's mysterious outbreak of "legionnaire's disease."

The epidemiologist collects data, looks for what we call "risk factors" (the biological or environmental circumstances that appear to make the development of a disease more likely) and tries to identify plausible cause and effect relationships. He or she does this on a large scale, often working with whole population groups (as opposed to individual patients), and may rely on statistics gathered by national or local governments, health and welfare agencies and educational institutions. This group of scientific students has done a great job in correlating heart disease and diet— a relationship that is now well accepted by nearly everyone. Some of the epidemiologists working on the heart studies saw similarities to the cancer problem, and they are now using their experience and renewed vigor to identify and attack risk factors in cancer. For many years now they have been studying worldwide cancer rates.

Cancer rates vary tremendously from one country to another.

This was puzzling for a while. We've known for a long time that cancer is not "contagious." But if one doesn't "catch" cancer, if it's not passed along from person to person within a certain locality, how to account for the fact that there's more of it in some places than in others? How to explain the low rate in primitive societies as opposed to the higher rates in the more technically advanced and affluent cultures? How to account for the fact that there are nearly three times as many cancer deaths in Scotland as in Mexico, and five times as many cancer deaths in Japan as in Thailand?

One theory was that these differences had to do with the genetic makeup of various populations. Some nationality groups, it was thought, might simply *inherit* a vulnerability to certain forms of the disease, while others remained fairly immune.

It was a rather shaky supposition from the start. Whatever the social and cultural dissimilarities, people living in different countries and even on different continents are biologically pretty much the same. True, hair color ranges from yellow to black, skin tones vary and noses and eyes take different shapes. But healthy human lungs, colons and livers function in exactly the same way the world over.

We know that though there is some validity to the concept of genetic immunity, it works only on an individual basis, not for whole population groups. We can say this with certainty because we've seen what had seemed to be genetic immunity disappear in a matter of years when members of a particular nationality group moved from one country to another.

The most striking example is provided by Japanese immigrants to the United States. Cancer rates in Japan are very different from what they are here. In Japan there is a relatively high incidence of stomach cancer and a fairly low incidence of cancer of the breast and colon. (We say of the Japanese that they are at "high risk" in terms of cancer of the stomach, and at "lower risk" for breast cancer and colon cancer.) Here in the United States, the situation is reversed: there is a high incidence of breast and colon cancer and a lower incidence of cancer of the stomach.

If the Japanese were so genetically constituted that they were just "naturally" more vulnerable to stomach cancer and less vulnerable to breast and colon cancer than people born in the United

States, we could expect their cancer risk pattern to remain the same no matter where they choose to live. But it doesn't work that way.

In a matter of years after moving to the United States Japanese immigrants begin to acquire the cancer risk pattern of people born in this country. Their incidence of stomach cancer begins to go down, while their incidence of breast and colon cancer goes up. The rate at which they acquire their new U.S. risk pattern depends on how rapidly they adopt the lifestyle of this country. Epidemiological studies such as the ones done with Japanese immigrants to the United States have knocked the national genetic immunity theory into a cocked hat. Something changes when people pack their bags and move from one country to another, but it's not their genes. It's their environment!

Following the environmental lead, epidemiologists in Japan and in the United States began sifting through factor after factor in an attempt to discover just which environmental influences might result in those changing cancer risk patterns. The one that correlates most closely with the changing risk patterns was found to be diet!

Just how different is the diet of the average Japanese from that commonly eaten on this side of the Pacific? To begin with, even taking into account that as a group they are somewhat smaller in stature than Americans, the Japanese subsist on far fewer calories. They consume about 5 percent less protein and, most significant of all, about 68 percent less fat. High-roughage vegetables account for a bigger proportion of their diet as compared with ours. Though the difference in carbohydrate consumption is small (351 grams a day in Japan versus 385 grams a day in the United States), the Japanese consume most of theirs in the form of rice.

Toshio Oisio, a consultant to the International Medical Foundation of Japan, tells us in a paper read at a symposium on nutrition in the causation of cancer that it is still not unusual for rice to make up from 50 to 60 percent of a person's diet in Japan. It's sometimes formed into balls and then baked until the outside is cooked to a glassy black hardness. Or it may be pounded into a cake which is dipped into sauce and charred in an oven or on a grill. The rice is often accompanied by something salty, such as soybean paste (miso) or sauce (shoyu), salty pickles or pickled fish, or shellfish or seaweed boiled with soybean sauce. Fish is frequently dipped in soy sauce and baked until the skin is blackened. The national preference for charred, salty food is apparent even in the way they prepare beefsteak (still a relatively new commodity in Japan) by first sprinkling it with soybean sauce and then grilling it over a charcoal fire until the outside surfaces are burned. One thing is certain about the Japanese diet: hamburgers, malts and french fries it's not.

Studies of Japanese immigrants living in Hawaii indicate a tendency to "Americanize" the diet. Typically, the Japanese in Hawaii begin to eat more fat, while their carbohydrate consumption drops off somewhat; a greater percentage of carbohydrates comes from sugar (35 percent in Hawaii compared to 20 percent in Japan). They also begin to cook differently, doing less baking and grilling to the charred state. This is still a long way from traditional American high-fat, high-protein, highly refined carbohydrate and low-roughage cuisine, but it's closer. And the closer the diet comes to the American norm, the more their cancer risk pattern looks like the one of native-born Americans.

That's not altogether a bad thing for the Japanese. In adopting an Americanized diet, they're trading in a lower risk of breast cancer and colon cancer for a lowered incidence of cancer of the stomach. The cure rate for stomach cancer is about 5 percent, while cure rates for both breast and colon cancers are approximately 10 times greater. In some ways the Japanese are worse off and in others better after they move here.

We're now carefully watching as changes take place in the risk pattern in Japan itself. We're all aware that for some years now Japan has been caught up in what can only be called the throes of Americanization. As the small island country becomes more and more Americanized, the Japanese diet is changing. Traditional eating habits continue to prevail; charred rice cakes and fish are still important, and the level of fat in the diet has stayed well below what most Americans consume. But some segments of the population are eating greater quantities of red meat, eggs, milk and milk products and less of the traditional food. As this change occurs, the incidence of stomach cancer in Japan is slowly tapering off while colon cancer, cancer of the breast and other typically American ailments—including heart disease—are on the rise.

But, you may still be wondering, why do we attribute these

changing cancer rates to diet? Isn't it just possible that other environmental factors are more important than food? Couldn't it be that the Japanese acquire a higher rate of colon and breast cancer when they move to Hawaii or the continental United States because of air and water pollution?

It could be, but it probably isn't. Let's not forget that the air and water in Japan's big industrial cities are at least as polluted as our own. In fact, people who move from, say, Tokyo to Hawaii or rural California are going from a highly polluted environment to areas that are relatively pollution free. Yet their cancer risk changes all the same.

It's a sad fact that so many of us have to live with air and water pollution. It goes without saying that we should make every effort possible to clean up the environment. Nevertheless, though pollution is ugly and unhealthy, where cancer is concerned it appears to be less important than the food we eat.

We know this because right here in the United States certain groups living side by side with the rest of us—breathing the same air and drinking the same water and thus exposed to the same environmental carcinogens—enjoy a much lower cancer rate than the population at large.

The Seventh-Day Adventists are a prime example. About 80 percent of the members of this religious group might be called "moderate" vegetarians. They eat eggs, milk, cheese and other dairy products, but no animal flesh. They stay away from coffee, drink very little tea and use condiments sparingly. Their fat intake is estimated to be about 35 percent less than the average American's and they consume a far greater amount of roughage. Seventh-Day Adventists don't smoke or drink as a rule, but even their mortality rate from cancers *not* related to smoking and drinking is from 30 to 50 percent lower than mortality rates for the population at large.

Thirty to fifty percent less cancer! And again, it looks as though the factor that sets this group apart from other Americans is diet.

Many of us with a professional interest in health and preventive medicine believe that there's a lot to be learned from the Seventh-Day Adventists. In chapter 4 we're going to take a closer look at them and the way they live. It's because of the Seventh-Day Adventists and groups like them, whose eating habits *and* cancer rates are different from those of other Americans, that we've come to accept the concept that the food we eat is a big factor in whether we will or won't be victims of cancer.

Perhaps you've noticed that so far I've spoken of food as a cancer *factor,* not a cause. That's because we have little reason to believe that diet alone is responsible for cancer or that particular foods are carcinogenic. The theory is not so scarifying or simple.

From 10 to 20 percent of all cancers are thought to be due to viruses, radiation or predisposing diseases. The other 80 to 90 percent are believed to be triggered by exposure to chemical carcinogens in the environment. (The term environment here is used in its broadest sense and includes the air we breathe and the water in our lakes, streams and oceans, our clothing, and all the physical materials with which we come into contact in our homes and on the job—including food.)

Many of these carcinogens have already been identified. There are undoubtedly many, many more of which we're not yet aware. It may not even be important to identify every carcinogenic substance in the environment, however. Most of them are present at such low levels that cancer does not result from exposure to them unless the host—that's you or me—is vulnerable. If we could find out more about how to lessen our vulnerability, we might in the long run be better off than if we were able to track down each potential carcinogen with an eye toward either eliminating it or staying away from it. (In fact, it would be impossible to eliminate or avoid all of them, since some low-level carcinogens, as we will see later in this book, are products of our own bodies' functioning.)

The important thing is: we've all been exposed to carcinogenic chemicals during our lives, but we don't all get cancer. For cancer to be the ultimate result of exposure to a carcinogen, either the exposure must be to a very large amount of the substance or some other factor or set of circumstances must have made the body vulnerable to the carcinogen. That's where diet comes in. We believe that the kind of food people eat day in and day out is an important modifying factor. It can make the body more vulnerable to certain carcinogens so that cancer develops. Or it can protect against the disease.

Evidence accumulated through experiments made with laboratory animals lends plausibility to the theory. These experiments are usually done with a control group of animals and a test group. The control group is fed normally. The test group gets a diet that is different in numbers of calories; or in the percentage of fats, proteins or carbohydrates; or in vitamin and mineral content. After a predetermined period has passed, a potent carcinogen is administered to both groups. Researchers have discovered that such dietary manipulations have a definite effect on the number of tumors the animals develop. In fact, we have no doubt at all that tumor incidence in animals depends to a large degree on how they have been fed.

Yes, we always need to keep in mind that information obtained from animal experiments may not be applicable to people. Though there are many biological similarities between human beings and the test animals that are used most frequently (rats, mice, dogs and monkeys), there are also some important differences. But we can begin to take animal data more seriously when it correlates with what is observed in groups of people. In the case of diet and cancer, epidemiological studies and animal studies reinforce each other. Each indicates that eating habits influence the incidence of cancer.

Both kinds of evidence are extremely valuable in trying to discover what causes disease. Medical investigators, doing individual case study work, are currently gathering information that may lead to a third kind of evidence. In the individual case study approach, information is collected on a patient's previous illnesses, health of parents and other family members, occupation, general background and lifestyle. The resulting case history is matched against the history of a healthy person of similar age and background. In this way we can get a better idea of who is most likely to have a particular disease and why.

Case study work was of the utmost importance in making the connection between cancer and smoking. Unfortunately the method doesn't lend itself well to testing theories about diet and cancer. If you're a smoker, you know it. You can tell an investigator approximately how many years you've been smoking and how many cigarettes or packs you smoke per day. Food is different. Most people can't remember with any degree of accuracy the specific foods they've eaten over a long period of time. (If you doubt it, see if you can recall all that you've eaten during the past week.) Of course, a person may be able to answer an investigator in generalities and say that he or she "likes meat," or eats "a lot" of meat. But this hardly adds up to sound scientific data.

Evidence based on good case study work would be the final proof that diet is indeed a major factor in the development of many of our most virulent forms of cancer. Even in its absence, however, we have enough to go on to make a strong case for the connection.

3

Overnourished—and Cancer Prone

Have you noticed that old people—really old people—tend to be a slender, wiry-looking lot? Some of them are downright scrawny. I don't know about you, but I for one have seen few extremely fat octogenarians.

It's no coincidence. We know that eating too much of the wrong kinds of food is a factor in the development of heart disease, diabetes and a host of other serious ailments that can lead to an early grave. Now we believe that certain dietary excesses—overnourishment is what I prefer to call it—are a key factor in the development of some kinds of cancer.

What's overnourishment? Well, to begin with, it isn't necessarily the same as obesity. The fat person may be overnourished (and probably is). But *the overnourished person isn't necessarily fat.* Maybe the best way to define the concept is to say that in overnourishment the body is consistently supplied with too much of certain kinds of food—more fats, protein and highly refined carbohydrates than it actually needs to function normally and well. More, in fact, than it may be able to handle.

Remember, human beings didn't always eat the way the majority of Americans and western Europeans do now. It's widely accepted that the first people existed mainly on a diet of fruits and nuts and whatever other vegetation was deemed edible. Meat and other animal products entered the picture at some point, but no one can say exactly when. In any event, it's unlikely that meat was an important part of the human diet until recently (speaking in evolutionary terms). Certainly throughout recorded history only the privileged classes could look forward to meat on a daily basis. The lower orders—and they were always the majority—subsisted mainly on the starchy vegetables (wheat or rice or corn or taro or potatoes, depending on where they lived), plus, for variety, whatever else they could manage to grow, scavenge or buy. The situation remains the same in many countries even today.

We know, too, that over the thousands and thousands of years since the first humanoid creatures roamed the earth in search of food, abundance was always the exception. Most of our ancestors had to struggle to get enough to eat, so the human body evolved in ways that enabled it to make the most efficient use of whatever bits and shreds of nourishment were available.

Then, suddenly (again in evolutionary terms) in our part of the world, the situation was reversed. Our systems, designed to wring the last molecule of sustenance from a meager food supply, suddenly had to cope with plenty. And it wasn't plenty of the old vegetarian foods to which the body had adapted itself over millions of years. It was plenty of a *different* kind.

Enormous technological advances in growing, processing, preserving, packaging and transporting foodstuffs of all varieties triggered drastic changes in our eating habits. Once you had to be wealthy or live on a farm to have eggs and bacon for breakfast whenever you wanted them. Once you had to bake all day (or employ servants who would do it for you) in order to have cake or pie for dessert. Now all you need is the frozen food counter at the supermarket. In short, nowadays you don't have to be rich to eat rich. And eating rich means cream in your coffee, butter on your bread and a chop or steak (or at least meat loaf) on your plate alongside the mashed potatoes.

While the change in eating habits didn't take place overnight, it did happen within the last hundred years or so, and in evolutionary terms this is even less than overnight. Our digestive organs and our metabolism (the complex physical and chemical processes by which energy is created and used within the body) haven't had time to adapt to the abrupt switchover from one kind of diet to another. Ordinarily I dislike analogies that compare the human body to a machine, but in this instance it's fair to say that eating the diet that prevails in the United States and other affluent countries of the West is like trying to run our low-combustion Stone Age bodies on twentieth-century jet fuel. After a while, oversupplied with too much of the wrong kind of fuel, the mechanism rebels. Many kinds of cancer, we believe, are manifestations of the mechanism gone haywire.

Consider this: researchers have repeatedly demonstrated that it's easier to induce tumors in laboratory animals that are purposely overfed, especially when the added calories come in the form of fats and proteins.

It works the other way around as well. Out of all the cancer studies done with animals, some of the most startling results have come from experiments in which the animals were placed on special diets. In one series of tests, for example, the goal was to see how calorie restriction would influence the development of mammary tumors. Fifty mice were fed the customary laboratory food mixture in the usual amounts. They were the control group. Fifty other mice were fed the same kind of food, but only half as much of it. A potent carcinogen, one known to produce mammary tumors in mice, was administered to the animals in both groups. Twenty mammary tumors developed in the control group—just about what the researchers expected. There was only one tumor in the calorie-restricted group.

Results were similar in other studies designed to see what would happen when the amount of fats and carbohydrates in the animals' diet was reduced. In one series of tests, where the goal was again to find out how diet would affect the development of mammary tumors, tumors developed in 100 percent of the control group of mice, but in only 15 percent of the mice on carbohydrate- and fat-restricted diets.

When animal experiments yield results as startling as these, we have to pay attention. We have to figure out how much applies to human beings. We have to review what we know about the distribution of the disease and see if there are any epidemiological parallels.

One thing seems clear at the outset: the relationship of cancer to calorie intake is not a direct one. We know, for example, that laborers and athletes, who may eat anywhere from five to seven thousand calories a day but use them all up in physical activity, are no more cancer prone than sedentary types who consume in the neighborhood of three to four thousand calories a day. In other words, just eating a lot doesn't seem to invite cancer—not if all those additional calories are burned off.

But what about eating a lot and getting fat? Here it would seem that we're getting closer to something important. A fascinating study was carried out several years ago by Dr. Albert Tannenbaum. He was able to gather insurance records dating from 1887 to 1921. Wherever possible, he noted the weight of the insured at the time the policy was issued and matched that information with the group's cancer mortality statistics. He found that men who were overweight by 25 percent or more had a cancer mortality rate that was approximately 30 percent higher than the men whose weight was normal or slightly below normal. There was also a gradient: the more overweight the man, the more likely he was to die of cancer.

The data appeared in Dr. Tannenbaum's textbook *Physiology of Cancer,* published in 1959. To date there have been no good follow-up studies verifying obesity as a risk factor in the development of most kinds of cancer. With the exception of cancer of the uterus and cancer of the kidney in women, we can't just come out and say that the fatter a person is, the greater his or her cancer risk, because Tannenbaum's study is the only one that supports the statement.

If consuming large numbers of calories isn't a factor, and if obesity may only be a factor some of the time, then why do we not dismiss those animal studies as irrelevant to cancer in human beings?

Because epidemiologists have discovered that wherever people eat a high-fat, high-protein diet that is also rich in highly refined carbohydrates and low in roughage, there is also a high incidence of certain kinds of cancers. These are the cancers described by Dr. John Berg of the Cancer Epidemiology Research Center at the University of Iowa as cancers of "affluent nutrition." They include cancer of the breast, colon, uterus, prostate, ovary and pancreas.

In analyzing international studies, we find that breast cancer correlates with a high national per capita intake of fat and protein. Colon cancer correlates with a high per capita consumption of meat and fat.

Cancer of the prostate correlates with high meat, fat, milk and sugar intake.

The evidence against fat in particular is especially strong, as a glance at graphs 3 and 4 will indicate. In fact, the correlation between breast cancer, colon cancer and fat intake on a country-by-country basis is positively breathtaking.

It's not just overeating, then, but overeating certain kinds of foods—especially fats and proteins—that increases the risk of certain cancers.

But just what does "overeating" mean in this context? How do you measure it? Those are difficult questions to answer specifically. Your individual needs for almost every vital nutrient vary depending on how old you are and whether you're a man or a woman—and if you're a woman, on whether you're pregnant or breast-feeding. Your activity level and the general state of your health are also important.

We do know that in this country the average person consumes something like 155 grams of fat per day. That's about 43 percent of the total diet. The Japanese, however, demonstrate that human beings can get by very nicely on about one-third that amount, 42 grams of fat per day, without suffering from fat deficiency ailments (if indeed there are such diseases). If your body can maintain itself on a lot less fat—or a lot less of any substance—than it usually gets, I think we can safely assume that what it usually gets is too much.

It's the same with protein. Nutritionists have established that a moderately active man weighing about 154 pounds needs something like seventy grams of protein a day to stay in good health, while a 123-pound woman needs about sixty grams of protein daily. (Pregnant and lactating women need more.) The actual amount of protein we get varies from person to person and from day to day, but nutrition studies tell us that the average daily protein intake of people in this country runs to nearly one hundred grams. That's almost 30 percent more than what the average 154-pound man needs and almost 40 percent more than the require-

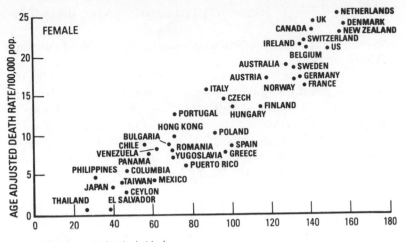

3. Correlation between per capita consumption of dietary fat (34) and age-adjusted mortality from breast cancer in different countries (72). The values for dietary fat are averages for 1964 to 1966 and those for cancer mortality are for 1964 to 1965, except in a few cases where data were available only for 1960 to 1961 or 1962 to 1963.

Reprinted by permission from "Experimental Evidence of Dietary Factors and Hormone-Dependent Cancers" by Kenneth K. Carroll, in *Cancer Research*, Vol. 35, p. 3379.

4. Bowel Cancer Mortality and Dietary Fat and Oil Consumption

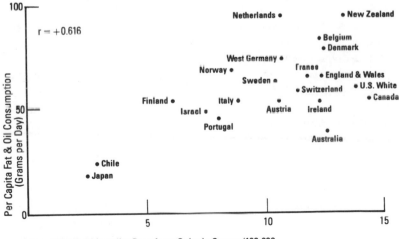

Source: Wynder, 1975.

Reprinted by permission from "The Epidemiology of Large Bowel Cancer" by Ernest Wynder, in *Cancer Research*, Vol. 35, p. 3389.

ments of a 123-pound woman. Again, we have a situation of chronic oversupply.

In the past seven years we've heard a great deal about the importance of protein in maintaining good health. Protein is often emphasized over all other nutrients. Diet books and articles about nutrition in the popular magazines are forever enjoining us to make' sure that we get "plenty" of it—usually without specifying what "plenty" or even "enough" of it might be. In reading this material, it's easy to get the feeling that the more protein you eat, the better off you're going to be.

These same books and articles often include a listing of prime sources of protein. Invariably red meat heads the list. (I've met some otherwise knowledgeable people who actually believe that meat is the *only* good source of protein.) The list usually goes on to include poultry, fish and other animal products such as eggs, milk and cheese.

No doubt about it, those foods *are* high in protein. But it's time we started questioning the notion that only good can come of eating unrestricted amounts of protein. We certainly have to reexamine the idea that red meat and other animal products are the most valuable sources of protein for human beings. It's possible to get plenty of protein and at the same time cut back on consumption of animal products. It's probably highly desirable to do so. As we've seen, wherever there is "affluent nutrition" there is also a high incidence of certain kinds of cancer.

Just what happens to our bodies when they are subjected to chronic nutritional overload? That for the moment is the sixty-four-billion-dollar question.

One obvious consequence of overnourishment is gaining weight and getting fat. But just as not all dietary deficiencies lead to emaciation, we believe that not all dietrary excesses lead to obesity. For example, the man with atherosclerosis, his arteries narrowed and partially blocked by fatty deposits, isn't necessarily overweight. Nevertheless, a diet high in saturated fats probably contributed to his condition.

Obesity, then, is only one response to overnutrition. Where one person gets fat, another may increase his or her metabolism to the point where nutritional excesses can be burned off. Undoubtedly there are other responses. Perhaps overnutrition results in the delivery of increased amounts of nutrients to specific organs or groups of cells. If increased fuel stimulates increased metabolic activity on a cellular level, some of that activity may become deranged. Rapid, abnormal cell growth—cancer—may be the result.

We know that in animals increased fat intake increases the production of certain hormones and that at least one hormone—estrogen—is a low-level carcinogen. Cholesterol, too, which is not only taken in with certain foods but produced in our bodies as well, is a low-level carcinogen. (We'll be taking a closer look at estrogen and cholesterol later in this book.)

Another theory has to do with animal fats and proteins and their effect on the body's immune system. All substances alien to the body are "checked out" by the immune system and either accepted as harmless or rejected and, if possible, destroyed. Food is readily identified and accepted by the immune system.

There's good reason to believe that small numbers of cancer cells are formed in the body every day. So long as the immune system is strong and on the alert, it is able to detect those cancer cells and do away with them before they can reach tumor proportions. However, the chemical makeup of some of the more complex animal fats and proteins we eat may not be greatly different from the chemical makeup of cancer cells produced by the body. Large amounts of these fats and proteins presented to the immune system may confuse and desensitize it, making it less well able to identify cancer cells, and allowing them to proliferate.

There is evidence to support each of these theories about what happens when our bodies are subjected to chronic nutritional overload—overnourishment, in other words. Whether time and future research will validate them remains to be seen. What we do know right now is that affluent eating habits are a risk factor in certain kinds of cancer. We also know that some groups in our population—well fed but *not* overnourished—enjoy a much lower cancer rate than the rest of us. Let's take a look at one of them.

4

The Seventh-Day Adventists: Living Proof That Diet Makes a Difference

I'm not interested in changing anyone's ideas about religion. I'm a Presbyterian myself, but I don't much care how my neighbors worship or whether they worship at all. I do care about health, and when one particular group—be it a religious group or a nationality group (or a singing group for that matter)—demonstrates a remarkably good health record over the years, I think we have to find out more about them. I think this applies even more when that group has a low incidence of cancer. If they're doing something right—or better than the rest of us—we should find out what it is so that we can emulate them.

In chapter 2 I mentioned that the Seventh-Day Adventists, a Protestant religious sect, have a cancer rate very much lower than that of the rest of our population. I also mentioned that we believe their low cancer rate can be explained by their eating habits. It has been suggested that some other aspect of the Adventist lifestyle might account for their relative freedom from malignancy, but most of those other aspects have been looked into. They're significant, but none explains all the cheerful statistics. Diet *is* important!

Religious beliefs and dietary differences aside, Adventists live very much like most other people in the United States. They don't sequester themselves in remote rural areas. Their lives are not ascetic and otherworldly. For the most part they are very much in the mainstream of twentieth-century American society. Many Adventists live in big cities; others reside in suburbs and small towns. A few do live in the country. But wherever they live, they drink the same water, wear the same kinds of clothes, drive cars on the same highways, watch the same tv shows and shop in the same supermarkets and department stores as their neighbors. They also hold many different kinds of jobs. In short, they're exposed to the same wide range of environmental carcinogens as other Americans.

They are, on the average, more highly educated. The percentage of Adventists with college degrees is twice the percentage of people with college degrees in the general population. At one time researchers wondered whether education might somehow be a factor in the Adventists' lower cancer rate. But no, as it turns out, schooling has nothing to do with it.

We say this because epidemiological studies clearly indicate that in the population as a whole there's no appreciable difference between the cancer rates of college graduates and non–college graduates. But when compared with control groups of men and women with identical educational backgrounds, the Adventists' cancer rate is far lower.

Another persuasive observation is that people who convert to Adventism as adults also tend to have less cancer than the population as a whole. In other words, one needn't be born and raised in the faith in order to acquire the Adventists' lower cancer rate. One need only adopt certain aspects of their lifestyle. Just as migrants from one country to another finally assume the cancer risk pattern of their new homeland, converts to Adventism trade their original risk pattern for the risk pattern of the Adventists!

If the Seventh-Day Adventists' protection from cancer is unrelated to high levels of education, if it can be acquired after childhood simply by adopting the Adventist lifestyle which is so similar to that of other Americans—save for diet and the avoidance of alcohol and tobacco—then it's logical to assume that eating habits and avoiding alcohol and tobacco are crucial.

Very few developments would be more gratifying to doctors than to learn that all smokers had kicked the habit. The same goes for drinking to excess. I'd be the last one to minimize the health hazards of these practices. But this is a book about cancer and nutrition. So I want to emphasize again that Seventh-Day Adventists enjoy a lowered cancer rate even with regard to those forms of the disease that are *unrelated* to smoking and drinking. Compared to other nonsmoking, nondrinking segments of the population, the Adventists still come out way ahead with a cancer mortality rate that is from 30 to 50 percent lower!

There aren't many Adventists in the Midwest, where I live, but a small group of them supports one of the local hospitals in Kansas City. In trying to find out more about the group and how they live—and most important, how they eat—I got in touch with the chaplain of the hospital, Chaplain Eldon Smith. Time spent with Chaplain Smith and his family was not only valuable to me in researching this book but enjoyable as well.

At our first meeting, Chaplain Smith, a genial, balding man of medium height—but rather too expansive of girth—expressed his pleasure at my interest in the Adventists. However, he wasn't the least bit surprised at my reasons for contacting him. Like many other Adventists I've met since then, the chaplain is aware of and highly gratified by the fact that the Adventist lifestyle is beginning to attract the attention of cancer researchers around the world. He was pleased to fill me in on some of the basic facts about the Adventists.

Worldwide there are about 2.5 million members of the church. About 500,000 of them live in North America, their greatest concentration being in southern California. The church was organized in 1863 by a small group of men and women who were convinced that the Second Coming of Christ was near at hand. Now as then, they base their faith and practice wholly on the Bible, which they interpret literally. Profoundly interested in maintaining good health, they believe that God's original prescriptions for vigorous health and longevity were recorded in the Bible and that it only remains to us to follow them and reap the benefits.

Chaplain Smith pointed out some of the Biblical passages that have shaped the Adventists' diet. In Genesis, for example, God says to Adam, "I have given you every herb bearing seed, which is upon the face of the earth, and every tree in which the fruit of the tree yields seed; to you, it shall be for meat." The Adventists interpret this to mean that the very first diet of humankind consisted entirely of fruit, nuts and grain—the seed-bearing parts of the plant.

After Adam was exiled from the Garden of Eden for disobedience, that first diet was modified and he was given permission by God to eat other parts of plants—stalks, leaves, roots—as well. Vegetables were added to the diet.

An account of God's granting the first permission to use animals as food is also found in the Bible. The passage recounts how, a millennium after Adam, the great Flood in Noah's time destroyed all vegetation. God said then that "every moving thing that livest shall be meat for you, even as the green herb have I given you all things." This was not to be taken as carte blanche permission, for there were qualifications: 1. The flesh to be eaten must first have been drained of all blood. 2. Only clean animals were to be used for food. 3. Animals were not to be killed unnecessarily.

The Seventh-Day Adventists' definition of "clean meat" is derived from the same Biblical text that governs Jewish dietary law. The details are to be found in Leviticus, chapter 11. To simplify, it was permissible to eat cud-chewing animals with cloven hooves, animals with fins and scales, and fowls of the nonscavenger type.

Since the Bible explicitly states that God gave humankind permission to eat the flesh of animals, the Adventists don't consider meat eating to be a sin. Their reasons for avoiding meat are based entirely on considerations of health and longevity.

In the Bible the human lifespan until the time of the Flood is said to have been approximately 960 years. After the Flood, when meat eating was permitted, lifespans mentioned in the Bible shrank to a mere 180 years or so. After the Biblical era, as men and women strayed farther and farther from the guidelines originally handed down by God, human life expectancy was abbreviated even more drastically until it had dwindled to a mere 30–35 years in the Middle Ages—since which time there has been only modest improvement.

The Adventists act—or shall we say eat—on the premise that the ideal diet for health and longevity was originally handed down by God. Meat eating was a compromise necessitated by the Flood.

Most Seventh-Day Adventists are what we call "lacto-ovo-vegetarians"—which means that though they abstain from eating animal flesh, they do drink milk and eat eggs and dairy products such as cheese. (By contrast, the true or pure vegetarian touches no food of animal origin. Another subcategory, the "vegens," go several steps further still; not only do they not eat anything of animal origin, they also go to great lengths to avoid using articles made of leather or fur or bone whose manufacture requires killing an animal.)

Adventists drink little if any coffee and tea and limit their use of spicy condiments. Many Adventists, though not all, avoid highly refined foods such as commercially prepared cakes, pastries and white bread.

Much of the high percentage of fat in the standard American diet comes from meat. By avoiding meat the Adventists typically consume about 25 percent less fat than the rest of us. They make up for meat by their far greater consumption of grains, nuts, fruits and vegetables. Thus, their diet is almost 50 percent higher in roughage than that of other Americans.

As we've seen, there are worldwide country-by-country correlations between overnourishment—the high-fat, high-protein, low-fiber diet—and certain kinds of cancer. These cancers—cancer of the breast, colon, uterus, ovary and prostate—are precisely the ones for which the Adventists have lower cancer rates than the rest of us.

Dr. Roland L. Phillips of Loma Linda University in California (an Adventist himself) offers several explanations as to how and why lacto-ovo-vegetarianism protects one against cancer.

For one thing, a diet low in fat and cholesterol may prevent the formation of large amounts of certain digestive chemicals that appear to make the colon more vulnerable to cancer.

A lower intake of fats and proteins may account for the fact that there is less obesity in Adventist women than in the general female population and also may influence hormonal output throughout life. These factors may explain the Adventists' lower incidence of breast cancer and cancer of the uterus and ovary.

Lower fat and protein intake may also make the body less susceptible to chemical carcinogens in the environment, in the same way that test animals on fat- and protein-restricted diets develop fewer tumors when exposed to carcinogens than control animals on nonrestricted diets.

Infrequent use of coffee might have something to do with the Adventists' reduced bladder cancer risk.

A high intake of vegetables, especially "cruciferous" vegetables (we'll have more to say about them later) and other vegetables rich in vitamins C and A, may protect against certain chemical carcinogens. (Animal tests indicate that both vitamins C and A are protective, although *excessive* amounts of A are dangerous and actually seem to promote tumor incidence.)

Finally, if you remember, we believe that the body's immune system may be somehow negatively influenced by the ingestion of large amounts of animal fats and proteins. By not eating meat, the Adventists may be keeping their immune systems more alert to small early clusters of tumor cells and thus better able to defend against cancer. This last, Dr. Phillips believes, may be a particularly fruitful area for future investigation. He and others suspect that the Adventists' across-the-board reduced cancer risk may be more indicative of particularly strong immunological defenses than of simple lack of exposure to potential carcinogens.

(I'm aware that some of the concepts touched on by Dr. Phillips may be unfamiliar to you. Many of these concepts will be taken up at greater length in the chapters that follow.)

Regardless of what the final verdict on some of these theories may be, it's obvious that the Adventists are doing something right and that something right has to do with the food they eat. But just what kind of food is it? What does one find on the Adventist table at breakfast, lunch and dinner? In response to my further questioning, Chaplain Smith invited me and my wife, Ruth, to join his family for dinner.

When we arrived, Chaplain and Mrs. Smith met us at the door and immediately led us to a table already spread with an array of appetizing dishes.

First we had a tropical punch made by blending bananas, orange juice, pineapple and Sprite. There were finger foods—vegetable sticks (carrots and celery) and whole wheat sticks. Then we were served oatmeal patties and baked sweet potatoes seasoned with apricot juice and walnuts. It was all delicious, even the dishes that were unfamiliar to Ruth and me. The two of us were particularly interested in some meat substitutes. Chaplain Smith told us they were called "meat analogs," such as chicken or beef analog.

We tried some of the chicken analog and found the taste and texture very good.

The meat analogs are made principally of highly refined soy or gluten (wheat) protein. Their texture is meatlike, and their flavors, though not actually duplicating the meat they're supposed to fill in for, are pleasant. They're extremely low in fat but add very little in the way of roughage to a meal. These analogs are about as close to eating meat as the Smiths ever come. Although somewhat less expensive than meat, these analogs are more difficult to find. Which is why some analogs, such as gluten, are made at home. A few are carried in supermarkets. Others need to be purchased in specialty stores such as those specializing in vegetarian diets or health foods.

After dessert of fresh fruits, the Smiths brought out a list of menus which they'd thoughtfully compiled for me. The list is representative of what the Smiths and other Adventists might eat over the course of a week. Take a look and see how it compares with the kind of food you and your family ordinarily have.

DAY #1

Breakfast: Granola cereal
Canned or fresh fruit
Milk

Lunch: Corn chowder
Fruit salad
Whole wheat bread
Milk

Dinner: Mock meatballs (made with beef analog) and
spaghetti
Tossed salad
Garlic bread
Fruit drink

DAY #2

Breakfast: Oatmeal
Fresh or canned fruit
Milk

Lunch:	Noodles Tossed salad Lemonade
Dinner:	Carrot roast Mashed potatoes and gravy Cucumber salad Fruit punch

DAY #3

Breakfast:	French toast with fruit Nuts Milk
Lunch:	Oatmeal patties Green beans Molded carrot and pineapple salad Milk
Dinner:	Baked rice with chicken analog Carrot sticks and olives Rye bread Gelatin dessert with pears

DAY #4

Breakfast:	Poached egg on whole wheat toast Banana Orange juice
Lunch:	Kidney bean soup Hot corn bread Apple cider
Dinner:	Tamale loaf Creamed peas Tomato salad Whole wheat bread Milk

DAY #5

Breakfast: Grilled sausage substitute with peach halves
Bran muffins
Milk

Lunch: Fruit soup (made with fresh fruits in summer, dried fruits in winter)
Nuts
Cottage cheese
Whole wheat bread

Dinner: Lentil roast
Noodles
Creamed asparagus
Lettuce with dressing
Whole wheat bread
Milk

DAY #6

Breakfast: Cottage cheese loaf (Recipe is on page 275)
Breakfast shake (orange juice, bananas and strawberries whipped to a froth in a blender)
Milk

Lunch: Chili (made with textured vegetable protein) served over corn chips
Lettuce, tomato, onion and shredded cheese salad
Lemonade

Dinner: Dinner rounds (canned textured vegetable protein)
Scalloped potatoes
Green beans
Carrot and apple salad
Fruit drink

DAY #7

Breakfast: Fruit dumplings (made with biscuit mix, chopped nuts, raisins, etc.)
Half grapefruit
Milk

Lunch: Cottage cheese loaf
Baked potato
Green beans with almonds or Bacos
Celery and carrot sticks
Tomato juice

Dinner: Creamed chicken analog on toast
Peas
Sliced tomatoes
Cranberry sauce
Milk

It occurred to me after reading this list that eating out might be a problem for the Adventists. I asked Chaplain Smith how he and his family fared at non-Adventist banquets, luncheons and other social or business functions where meat was sure to be served. Did the Smiths ever deviate from their accustomed eating habits in order to be sociable? Did they ever have to compromise just to get enough to eat?

The answer was no to both questions. According to Chaplain Smith, the Adventists do not feel they are being ungracious or impolite in declining food they feel strongly about not eating. Neither do they make any fuss about it. Instead, they simply eat around the meat—which is usually the entrée—and fill up on salad or other side dishes. "But," Chaplain Smith added, "traveling can be a problem. Sometimes it's downright impossible to find restaurants and cafeterias with good vegetarian dishes on the menu."

Then he told me about the time he and his family were traveling across central Europe. There were so few eating establishments serving the kind of food the Adventists eat that all through Austria, Germany and Luxembourg the family lived mainly on bread, cheese and candy bars. Even though this diet is acceptable to the

Seventh Day Adventists, it is high in fat and, as we will point out, the Seventh Day Adventist diet can be improved.

In a way, it figures. Luxembourg, of all countries for which figures are available, has the highest cancer rate.

At home that night Ruth and I talked about the evening. We'd enjoyed the Smiths. And much to our surprise we'd enjoyed the food. Midwesterners that we are, the meatless meal is still something of a novelty to us. But after visiting the Smiths and sampling their food, we felt that it would be no great hardship to live on such a diet. Certainly not if increased cancer protection was the reward for doing so.

But is lacto-ovo-vegetarianism the only way? Is giving up meat part of the price we must pay for bettering our chances of living cancer-free lives? I could do it, and I would, if I thought that were the case. But as the son of a Kansas cattle rancher the prospect of nothing but meatless meals is not a particularly happy one to me. And as a scientist I don't believe it's necessary to eliminate meat from the diet.

What's important is to avoid overnourishment. Even some of the Adventists, while doing a lot better than most of us, appear to be overnourished. Lacto-ovo-vegetarianism or no, Chaplain Smith was definitely overweight.

More important than cutting out meat entirely is to get along on less fat and somewhat smaller amounts of protein while at the same time increasing the amount of vegetables and other high-roughage foods. The fat factor is crucial, as we'll see in the next chapter. In fact, it's what the Anti-Cancer Diet is all about.

I'm not knocking vegetarianism. For those of you who want to try it I've included in this book important information about how to combine certain vegetable foods in order to get enough complete protein for good health. You'll also find some of Mrs. Smith's recipes in the meal-planning section. They're good-tasting, and whether you decide to switch to vegetarianism or not, they'll provide a nice change of pace for family meals.

I know, however, that if a food plan is going to be effective, people have to be able to really live with it. It seems to me that vast numbers of Americans would have trouble *living* with a diet that was entirely meatless. I know I would. That's why the Anti-

Cancer Diet as we've devised it includes meat of almost every kind and just about every other good thing that you're accustomed to. It's the *proportions* of the various food groups and the *way they're put together* that make the difference.

5

The Fat Factor

That fat *is* a factor in the onset of some common forms of cancer is well supported. What still isn't crystal clear is just *how* too much fat in the diet makes the body more vulnerable to the disease. To be sure, there are theories. Undoubtedly some of them will prove to be on target. But the ultimate proof isn't in yet—and it may be years, even decades, before it is.

In the meantime, says Dr. Ernst L. Wynder, president of the American Health Foundation, the relationship between fat and cancer puts us in the position of the owner of a china shop who enters the store only to find an angry bull amidst the wreckage of smashed cups, saucers and plates. Nobody actually saw the bull do the damage. We don't know whether he used his horns or his hoofs or lashed out with his tail. Yet there is the bull, and there is the smashed china, and rather than wait to find out exactly what happened, we'd be wise to get that animal off the premises.

Neither Dr. Wynder nor I nor anyone else suggests that fat alone causes cancer. It is not in itself carcinogenic. Rather, it is just what the title of this chapter states: a factor—perhaps one of two or three or even more factors which, when combined, make cancer not only likely but practically inevitable.

Some of the other factors may be such that we have no

control over them, although there is always the possibility that we will find ways to deal with them in the years to come. We might also be able to come up with efficient methods of arresting the disease in its early stages. Perhaps we will even find a cure. When that happens we will truly have licked cancer. But that's all in the future.

For now, we have a better handle on the *prevention* of the disease than we had before we had any inkling of the role played by diet—especially excess fat consumption—in its development. We *can* control what we eat. We *can* cut back on the amount of fat we take in. And when the fat factor is missing, those other less controllable factors are minus an ally. Without the fat factor it's going to be that much more difficult for them to gang up on us, making us sick from cancer.

From all I've learned during the course of researching this book, I would have to say that if just one single recommendation were to be made with regard to food—one sole lifesaving suggestion—it would be to restrict the amount of fat in your diet. The fat factor is that crucial.

To get a better understanding of how it operates, let's consider some of the cancers tied to affluent nutrition—one by one, starting with breast cancer.

Among the malignant diseases breast cancer is the third leading killer in this country, exceeded only by cancer of the lung and of the colon in the lives it takes each year. Here in the United States where a high-fat diet prevails, the mortality rate for breast cancer is 21.9 per hundred thousand in the population per year. In the Netherlands, where breast cancer is more common than in any other country and the mortality rate is 26.4 per hundred thousand, the female per capita fat consumption is 155 grams per day compared to 145 grams here.

In Japan, where fat makes up 30 grams per day, the mortality rate from breast cancer is a dramatically lower 4.4 per hundred thousand. (Other countries, Thailand, El Salvador and Sri Lanka (Ceylon) among them, also have low breast cancer mortality rates. However, we usually use Japan as an example because we know that statistical data from that country are meticulously gathered and reliable and that Japanese medical and scientific expertise are at least comparable to our own.)

A possible explanation for the great variation in the breast cancer rates of the countries mentioned has to do with the high-fat diet and its influence on hormones. (Hormones, as you may know, are chemical compounds manufactured by the endocrine glands; their function is to regulate the activity of other organs and tissues that are specifically receptive to them.)

We know that large amounts of fat in the diet modify the body's production of certain hormones. Among the hormones affected by excesses of dietary fat is a substance called prolactin. Prolactin is produced by the pituitary gland, located at the base of the brain, and it is primarily involved with breast tissue and the mammary glands. It is prolactin that stimulates the mammary glands to produce milk shortly after the birth of a baby.

As I've noted previously, it's easier to induce mammary tumors in animals on high-fat diets than in animals that are fed normally. One of the biochemical changes noted in the tumor-prone rats on a high-fat diet was an increase in the ratio of prolactin to estrogen in their bodies. (Estrogen as you no doubt know is another hormone, produced by the ovaries.)

Dr. Ernst Wynder reported to the U.S. Senate Select Committee on Nutrition about a study done with a group of nurses who voluntarily changed their eating habits to see if a low-fat vegetarian diet would affect the production of prolactin in their bodies. The study yielded impressive results: after only four weeks their levels of prolactin were decreased by from 40 to 60 percent.

Now what does this amount to? Circumstantial evidence, but extremely interesting nevertheless:

1. The production of prolactin appears to be increased by a high-fat diet.

2. A high ratio of prolactin to estrogen is found in test animals that develop mammary tumors.

3. Prolactin apparently can be reduced by decreasing the amount of fat in the diet.

It is the theory of Drs. Po-Chuen Chan and Leonard A. Cohen of the Naylor Dana Institute for Disease Prevention that a high ratio of prolactin to estrogen in the fluid and tissues of the breast greatly enhances a woman's chances for developing the disease. It is at the very least an intriguing theory, particularly since prolactin production can be modified and somewhat controlled by diet.

As I write this, researchers are in the process of finding out whether the chemical makeup of fluids in the breasts of Japanese women and other women who customarily consume low-fat diets is indeed measurably different from that of the breast fluids in women eating the standard American or western European diet. If it turns out, as they suspect it will, that the breast fluids of Japanese women, with their far lower risk of cancer of the breast, really do show lower levels of prolactin and some of the other breakdown products of fats and cholesterol, the theory will have been advanced several steps.

Chan and Cohen's theory would go a long way toward explaining what we call the "age incidence" patterns of breast cancer. You see, in the United States, the Netherlands and other countries where high-fat diets prevail and the breast cancer rate is correspondingly high, a woman's cancer risk tends to increase with age. An eighty-year-old woman is more likely to develop the disease than a seventy-year-old, who in turn has a greater risk than a sixty-year-old. In countries where the breast cancer rate is relatively low to begin with—such as Japan—a woman's risk increases until about the age of fifty, approximately the time when she reaches the menopause, and then tapers off.

The explanation would go something like this: the American woman consumes a high-fat diet throughout her life, and thus probably has a generally high periodic ratio of prolactin to estrogen throughout her fertile years. Menopause (and the decrease in estrogen production that comes with it) would exaggerate the ratio of prolactin to estrogen. Thus, her cancer risk would increase as estrogen production dropped off. The Japanese woman, consuming a low-fat diet from birth, would have relatively low levels of prolactin all during her life. Even with menopause and a decrease in estrogen production, the ratio of the two hormones would remain safer.

Other theories also implicate a high-fat, high-protein diet. But before we consider some of these lines of thinking, a bit more background on breast cancer is in order.

In chapter 2 I pointed out that Japanese immigrants to the United States acquire an increased risk of colon and breast cancer after living in this country for a while. The greater colon cancer risk is developed rather rapidly. It takes longer for breast cancer incidence to go up. In fact, it's often not the immigrant woman but her children who end up with an increased breast cancer risk. To put it another way, the Japanese woman who is in her thirties or forties when she arrives in this country will probably retain the lower Japanese breast cancer risk for the rest of her life. But a Japanese baby, born here or brought here in infancy, would—assuming her family immediately embraced American eating habits—have a breast cancer risk similar to that of an American girl of any parentage.

For this reason we believe that a high-fat, high-protein diet started early in life has serious implications for the future. In fact, for young children, a high-fat, high-protein diet amounts to a kind of "force feeding" for growth and rapid development, probably resulting in greater height and, in girls, an earlier menarche (first menstrual period).

And what's wrong with tallness and early sexual maturity? Not a thing. Except that both accompany an increased breast cancer risk.

The Netherlands, the country with the highest breast cancer rate in the world, has given us one of the most persistent and resourceful researchers in the field, Dr. F. de Waard. In 1974 Dr. de Waard came forward with data indicating a strong correlation between tallness, early menarche and breast cancer. He postulates that the tall woman, probably overnourished from birth, may experience an early menarche as a result of a disturbance in normal hormonal activity. Certainly, the height theory is consistent with the difference between the low cancer rate in Japan and the higher breast cancer rate in the United States and western Europe. However, among women within a given population—our own, for example—breast cancer is as apt to strike the petite as the willowy.

Early menarche *is* a risk factor in our population. In some studies the reported increase in the incidence of breast cancer is small but significant all the same. One recent set of data shows that when menarche occurs before age sixteen, there is a 1.8-fold increase in a woman's chances of developing the disease. (It's interesting that Seventh-Day Adventist women, who consume less fat than other women in the population, begin to menstruate at a somewhat later age than most American women—and also have a lower incidence of breast cancer.)

Other studies suggest that women who experience menopause at a later than usual age have a moderately increased breast cancer risk. One report indicates that women who reach the "change of life" at fifty-five or later have about twice the risk of women who do so before the age of forty-five.

The earlier the menarche and the later the menopause, the greater a woman's breast cancer risk. Menarche, menstruation and menopause—all are governed by the hormone estrogen, which is produced by the ovaries before menopause and afterward is manufactured in small amounts by tissue peripheral to the ovaries. It begins to look as though breast cancer is connected in some way with estrogen production and the length of time the ovaries produce it at peak capacity. This suspicion is buttressed by the fact that removal of the ovaries, resulting in a decrease in estrogen production, has brought about good therapeutic results in some breast cancer patients. Indeed, we've known for some time that estrogen is a weak carcinogen, that it produces tumors when administered to laboratory animals in large doses over long periods of time.

(Somewhat puzzling is that "exogenous" estrogen—estrogen not produced by the body but taken orally for therapeutic purposes—doesn't seem to increase a woman's chances for developing breast cancer. The estrogen in oral contraceptives places a woman at no greater risk, while estrogen replacement therapy to ease menopausal distress imposes only a slightly increased risk. This may happen because of the long latent period between the time of exposure to a carcinogen—in this case, estrogen—and the appearance of tumors. It could be that studies involving women who have taken exogenous estrogen have not accounted for this time lag. But no matter, we still *can't* feel completely at ease about the safety of estrogen therapy because we know that it increases the risk of another kind of cancer—cancer of the uterus.)

What does all of this have to do with diet? As I pointed out earlier, we know that a high-fat, high-protein diet influences the body's hormonal "milieu"—the amounts of the various hormones produced and the proportion of each to the others. Perhaps these changes make the body more vulnerable to environmental carcinogens. Or perhaps these changes render the hormones themselves carcinogenic, or more strongly carcinogenic (as may be the case with estrogen).

There is greater risk of breast cancer for women who have never borne a child. And the younger a woman is at the time she has her first baby, the smaller her risk. Women whose first pregnancies occur before the age of eighteen have only one-third the risk of women who wait until they're thirty-five to start a family. In fact, if pregnancy is going to be protective at all, it must occur before the age of thirty.

Another thing: only full-term pregnancies are protective; aborted pregnancies have no effect on cancer risk. On the other hand, a woman's cancer risk is not improved by having more than one child. Nor is breast-feeding a protective factor.

A history of breast cancer in the family is, of course, an added risk factor. This seems to indicate that though diet may be very important, so is an inherited vulnerability to the disease.

I offer all this information in the hope that women who are at greater risk—childless women and women whose mothers, grandmothers, aunts or sisters have had breast cancer—will be especially vigilant about self-examination and will also visit their doctors for frequent checkups.

Cancer of the uterus is another form of the disease that we believe is related to overnutrition. However, it is important to make a distinction between cancer of the body of the uterus (also called cancer of the endometrium, and the kind we're talking about here) and cancer of the cervix (the intravaginal extension or "neck" of the uterus).

Cancer of the cervix, the bigger killer of the two, is probably not related to fat intake, although another nutritional factor—vitamin A deficiency—may be significant in its development. Cancer of the cervix correlates with chronic infection of the cervix and sexual activity with many different partners. (The two may be part of the same phenomenon, since women who have intercourse with many different men will be exposed to a large variety of alien and potentially harmful organisms.)

Cancer of the uterus is a different matter. It's one of the two cancers which appear to be directly related to obesity (cancer of the kidney in women is the other). In fact a woman who is fifty pounds or more overweight is *ten times* as likely to become a victim of this disease as the woman of normal weight.

Diabetes is also related to uterine cancer. The kind of diabetes that develops in the mature woman—or man, for that matter—is frequently associated with obesity. Very often, "adult-onset" diabetes, as it is called, can be controlled or corrected by losing weight. Of all women in the population, the overweight diabetic is at highest risk for cancer of the uterus.

Interesting similarities exist between cancer of the uterus, cancer of the breast and cancer of the ovary. The woman who has had one of these cancers runs a greater risk of developing either or both of the others. As with cancer of the breast, there is a relationship between childbearing and cancer of the uterus. The woman who has never been pregnant has twice the risk as the woman with one child and three times the risk of the woman with five or more children. (In general it seems, cancer—except cancer of the cervix—tends to seek out nonmothers.)

A late menopause also increases risk. Women who experience menopause at age fifty-two or later are two and one-half times more likely to develop cancer of the uterus than women whose menopause occurs at age forty-five or before.

All of this leads to a conviction that hormone imbalances are a probable factor in cancer of the uterus, just as we suspect they are in breast cancer. Once again estrogen is high on the suspect list. Women who have taken exogenous estrogen for relief of menopausal symptoms have three times the risk of cancer of the uterus as other women their age. (Many doctors now feel that estrogen therapy should be restricted, that only the woman who has had a hysterectomy can safely take it.)

As for why obese women who have never taken the Pill or had any other kind of estrogen therapy should be at such great risk, let's not forget that a diet high in fat affects the body's hormonal milieu. It may be that overnourishment resulting in obesity alters the body's own estrogen output in ways that increase the hormone's carcinogenicity to the uterus.

Cancer of the ovary is the fifth leading cause of death by cancer for women. Between 1930 and 1955 the disease was on the rise. Since then, the mortality rate has remained stable.

This kind of cancer, for reasons no one yet understands, occurs somewhat more frequently in big-city dwellers and members of the higher socioeconomic groups. In New York, Jewish women are at higher risk than others. Ovarian cancer is more common in childless women, but not much.

Since the ovaries are the primary source of estrogen in premenopausal women, it's not surprising that cancer of the ovary appears to be connected with hormonal imbalance. Again there is a strong suspicion that too much fat in the diet sets the stage for its development.

Less is known about this kind of cancer than the other two mentioned so far, but it does share the same worldwide distribution pattern: it is less common in Japan and other countries where the population subsists on a relatively low-fat diet than in the United States and western Europe. Japanese immigrants to this country lose their low risk of this cancer, and as eating habits in Japan itself become more Westernized, there is a corresponding increase of the disease in that country.

Cancer of the prostate is another kind of cancer that we've been seeing more of over the past thirty years. It has also become more "curable." With treatment, approximately 50 percent of its victims now go on to live out their normal lives.

Some people are uncertain of the location of the prostate and its function. To set the record straight, the prostate is a firm glandular structure, somewhat smaller than an egg, located at the base of the urinary bladder and partially enfolding the urethra (the tube that leads from the bladder to the end of the penis and through which urine passes). A major function of the prostate is to supply ejaculatory fluid. When the prostate is enlarged, it tends to interfere with the passage of urine.

Not all enlargements of the prostate are due to malignancy; most men experience some nonmalignant enlargement of the gland in their later years and the condition is usually easily corrected by surgery.

The prostate is part of the male endocrine system, and cancer of the prostate—like cancer of the breast, uterus and ovary in women—is thought to have some connection with hormonal imbalances. Indeed, one way of treating the disease involves removal of the testicles (which produce sperm and the male hormone testosterone), just as treatment for female endocrine-related cancers may include removal of the ovaries (which produce eggs and the female hormone estrogen). Estrogen is often given as a therapy for cancer of the prostate.

Some seemingly inexplicable phenomena are associated with cancer of the prostate. One is its great rate of increase over the last three decades. In white American males this increase amounts to nearly 23 percent since 1947. More baffling still is the fact that there has been a *55.4* percent rise in black American males over the same period. As of now the disease is almost twice as common in blacks as in whites.

Nobody seems to know what to make of the racial discrepancy in the figures, which is apparent even when we compare blacks to whites doing the same kind of work or living in the same area. Smoking, alcohol and infectious diseases appear to have nothing to do with it, either. If the great increase in cancer of the prostate in black Americans were due to food additives, air pollution, water contamination or almost anything else we can think of, we would expect to see an equal increase in white males.

Among blacks the disease follows no socioeconomic or geographic patterns; it is found at about the same rate of incidence among northerners and southerners, men who live in rural areas and men who live in the cities. But cancer of the prostate does *not* appear to be on the rise in African blacks, nor is the black African as vulnerable to it. In fact, the American black is *seven times* more likely to develop the disease than the African black.

As with the other cancers discussed so far in this section, *international* variations do appear to follow a pattern. Cancer of the prostate is most common in Sweden and Switzerland, where mortality rates for the disease are slightly more than eighteen per hundred thousand in the population. (Black Americans have a mortality rate of twenty-eight per hundred thousand, but because the disease is seen far less frequently in white males, the total mortality rate in the United States is much lower.)

The lowest mortality rates for cancer of the prostate are seen in Thailand, the Philippines, El Salvador, Egypt and Hong Kong, and in Japan, where it is 1.93 per hundred thousand.

That worldwide distribution pattern is a familiar one to us by now: there is much less cancer of the prostate where a low-fat diet prevails and more of it where people consume the high-fat, high-protein, low-roughage diet of the affluent. But what about that exaggerated incidence of the disease in American blacks? Eating habits don't account for it, and for the moment we can only speculate as to its cause. Perhaps here is an instance where genetic factors do come into play. Perhaps American blacks are particularly hard hit by the disease because of a combination of a high-fat diet with some as yet unidentified inherited vulnerability. That American blacks are at a slightly higher risk in terms of other kinds of malignancies as well seems to bear this out. Improved statistical gathering on blacks plays an uncalculated role.

Cancer of the pancreas has a far less favorable cure rate than cancer of the prostate. But, like the latter, it's also on the rise. There has been a 30 percent increase in the incidence of cancer of the pancreas since 1945. This, plus its dismal cure rate, makes it imperative that we do all we can to identify and practice preventive measures.

The distribution of pancreatic cancer and its recent history are rather interesting: over the last thirty years we've seen a 20 percent increase in mortality from this form of cancer in white men and women. During the same interval the mortality rate for black males has increased by *30* percent, while the black female mortality rate has skyrocketed by *126* percent. In the past, the black woman enjoyed relative immunity from the disease; it is only since 1945 that her risk has been comparable to that of others in the population. This leads to speculation: either some factor that used to protect her is now absent or she has within the last thirty years been increasingly exposed to some carcinogen that the general population had always been exposed to in lesser or greater amounts. According to the latest statistics, the mortality rate from pancreas cancer for black women is 8.6 per hundred thousand—higher than the white woman's 6.5, but lower than the white male's 10.8 and much lower than the black male's 15.2.

The international profile for cancer of the pancreas differs from that of the other cancers discussed in this section. Polynesian natives of New Zealand and Hawaii have the highest rates in the world. The inhabitants of Nigeria and India have the lowest. Japan used to have a low rate of the disease, but we're seeing a rather dramatic upturn in its incidence there. The Japanese American has a risk approaching that of the American black, who ranks third in international incidence.

The low rate of the disease in Nigerian blacks, as opposed to the high rate in American blacks, plus the quickly changing rate in Japan suggest that environmental factors play an important role in the development of this kind of cancer.

It looks as though there's a connection with cigarette smoking. Smokers are about twice as likely to develop the disease as nonsmokers, and there is even evidence of what we call a "dose response gradient" indicating that the heavier the smoker, the greater his or her risk. In the past more men than women smoked, and they smoked *more*. This may explain why the incidence of cancer of the pancreas is higher in males. The increase in the number of women who smoke during the last couple of decades may explain the climbing incidence of the disease among white women. But the theory doesn't shed much light on why there has been such a spectacular increase in black women.

One study indicates a link between cancer of the pancreas and alcoholism. Other studies fail to corroborate this.

Tumors of the pancreas have been induced in laboratory animals with certain industrial chemicals. Therefore, some researchers believe that exposure to these chemicals, such as B napthylamine and benzidine, may be a factor. A study of the death certificates of a large number of chemists showed that a slightly greater percentage of them died as a result of cancer of the pancreas than we would expect to find in the population as a whole, but no specific chemical was indicted.

Diabetics definitely have an increased risk of cancer of the pancreas. Perhaps that is to be expected, since diabetes is the result of a malfunctioning pancreas.

Diabetes is a risk factor in only one other malignancy, cancer of the uterus. Cancer of the uterus, remember, like cancer of the breast and ovary, is thought to be related to disturbances of the hormone-producing endocrine glands. These disturbances appear to be connected with a high-fat diet. The pancreas also has an endocrine function: it secretes the hormone insulin directly into the bloodstream. All of this plus the fact that cellular changes in the tissues of the breast, ovary and uterus have been noted in patients with cancer of the pancreas make it impossible not to speculate that there are some very important relationships among these various cancers.

For now, the connection between eating habits and cancer of the pancreas is vague at best. We know that adult-onset diabetes can be controlled by keeping one's weight down, so diet may be protective in at least that one sense. We also know from studying the international distribution of the disease that some aspects of the American and western European lifestyle play a part in its development. Smoking and exposure to certain chemicals may be more important, but we still cannot completely rule out food.

6

The Case Against Cholesterol

In the last chapter we were concerned with dietary fat as a factor in the development of certain kinds of cancer. The whitish, tallowy substance rimming the edge of a pork or lamb chop, the grease that clings to the skin of a roast chicken, the liquid oil extracted from corn, peanuts and olives, and the solid shortenings such as lard, butter and margarine—all are fats. Based on the strong correlation between a high-fat diet and a high incidence of certain kinds of cancer, I'm going to recommend that you eat less of all types of fats. (Later in the book you'll find specific suggestions on how, and how much, to cut back.)

In this chapter we're going to focus on *cholesterol,* a fatlike substance that is found to a greater or lesser degree in all animal tissue, and for practical purposes *only* in animal tissue. But before we do, a few words about the relationship between cholesterol and saturated fats as well as unsaturated fats, all substances to which I'll refer in the pages that follow.

To begin with, all fatty substances are made up of atoms of carbon, hydrogen and oxygen linked together in various ways. Saturated fat molecules have as many hydrogen and oxygen atoms as they can possibly hold. In a sense they're "saturated" with hydrogen; it is hydrogen saturation that makes most of them solid at room temperature. Most highly saturated fats are of animal origin and thus have a close relationship to cholesterol. With the exception of coconut oil, a saturated vegetable fat, and one or two others, we can say that where there is saturated fat there is also cholesterol. A diet high in saturated fat tends to raise cholesterol levels in the blood—a situation that increases one's risk of heart disease.

There are fewer hydrogen atoms in molecules of unsaturated fats. They're "unsaturated" with hydrogen and are usually liquid at room temperature (corn oil margarine is an exception only because it has been partly hydrogenated to render it solid). Most highly unsaturated fats are of vegetable origin and thus contain no cholesterol. In addition, diets relatively high in unsaturated fat have been shown to produce a modest decrease in blood cholesterol, which is why the American Heart Association recommends that dietary fat contain more unsaturated than saturated fat as one way of reducing the risk of heart disease.

In the Anti-Cancer Diet we're going to make very little distinction between saturated and unsaturated fats. A diet high in either or both correlates with a high incidence of the cancers of affluent nutrition, so both saturated and unsaturated fats are undesirable from our point of view. But because saturated fats are so closely associated with cholesterol, and because there is mounting evidence that cholesterol is a factor in the development of colon cancer, I'm going to suggest that whenever the choice is up to you, you select unsaturated rather than saturated fats.

Cancer of the colon is a particularly prevalent form of the disease, second only to cancer of the lung in the lives it takes each year. In this country alone, almost forty thousand people will die of colon cancer this year. More will die the following year and even more the year after that. The mortality rate from cancer of the colon increased until 1945 and has been decreasing slowly, overall, since then (black males and females again being an exception). This is a result of improved diagnosis and treatment. However, though the cure rate is better, we are seeing more of the disease, especially among blacks, and we have to do all we can to prevent it. Lowering our cholesterol consumption might well be the key—or so recent studies show.

For example, there is a strong country-by-country correlation between the percentage of fat in the usual diet and the incidence of colon cancer. Generally speaking, the richer and more highly industrialized the country, the greater the incidence of colon cancer. But Denmark and Finland, though similar in terms of economic development, have quite different rates of cancer of the colon. The Danes, who are at considerably greater risk, consume a diet that is nearly 50 percent higher in fat than the Finns.

The United States has a higher rate of cancer of the colon than Puerto Rico despite geographical proximity and close political ties. The standard American diet is also higher in fat than the diet of most Puerto Ricans.

There are different rates of the disease for American blacks who live in the rural south and for those who live in northern cities. For many years *all* blacks were at less risk than whites, but this particular gap is closing rapidly. Many cancer experts believe that this increase among certain blacks is the result of integration into the mainstream of American life, with the better, more affluent standard of living—and diet—that that move implies.

In this country, the Seventh-day Adventists, who eat no meat and therefore consume less fat—and a great deal less cholesterol—have a colon cancer rate that is 50 percent lower than that of others in the population.

Finally, and this is *very* important, where coronary heart disease is a major health problem, so is cancer of the colon. As everyone knows by now, hypercholesterolemia—the presence of high levels of cholesterol in the blood—is a primary risk factor in heart disease. The person with an elevated cholesterol level is almost always urged to lower it by eating smaller amounts of animal fat. (He or she will also be told to stop smoking and start getting more exercise.)

All of these observations say something important about cancer of the colon, something indicating an extremely close connection between its development and the intake of dietary fat, particularly cholesterol.

Of course correlation is not the same as causation; it doesn't necessarily follow that people with certain eating habits have more cancer *because* of those eating habits. But let's also keep in mind that any theory about causation remains highly implausible if it is not backed up by correlation.

Dr. Wynder of the American Health Foundation and some of his associates believe that a diet too high in fat and cholesterol is the *primary* factor influencing whether a person will become a victim of colon cancer.

To understand their thinking, let's consider what happens to food once it's been chewed, swallowed, worked over by enzymes and other digestive chemicals in the stomach and passed on to the small intestine. At that point, a yellowish-green liquid called bile enters the picture.

The liver synthesizes bile from cholesterol. In fact, bile is a "breakdown product" of cholesterol. However, the liver doesn't need an outside supply of cholesterol from which to manufacture bile. It is perfectly capable of making enough cholesterol within itself to satisfy the body's needs. In a sense, then, *any* cholesterol that we take in with our food is excess.

Bile is not the only breakdown product of cholesterol. There are others, chemically similar to cholesterol, called neutral sterols. These are also processed through the liver.

In any event, the liver uses cholesterol to make bile, which is composed of various substances called bile acids, bile salts and neutral sterols. Bile is stored in the gall bladder. When partially digested fats make their way to the small intestine, bile is secreted via the biliary duct to mix with the fats and emulsify them, breaking them down into minuscule globules of fatty acids. Then the fatty acids and most of the bile products are absorbed by the small intestine and taken up by the bloodstream to circulate throughout the body. Bile products in the bloodstream eventually find their way back to the liver, where they are used again.

But small amounts of the bile acids and neutral sterols get passed on, along with unusable food waste, to the colon. The colon is inhabited by huge colonies of bacteria which do the final job of converting food waste and other waste into feces. Unfortunately some of these bacteria also go to work on the bile acids and neutral sterols, changing them into substances that are mildly carcinogenic.

Tests done with animals show that when bile acids are administered along with a known carcinogen, more tumors result than would have been expected if the carcinogen alone had been given.

We also know that the more bile acid is administered, the smaller the amount of the carcinogen needed for tumors to develop.

The theory, then, is that cancer is at least partially the result of these chemically changed bile acids coming into contact with the walls of the colon. Some researchers suspect that the cancer process is further speeded along by the presence of weak carcinogens in our food. Cholesterol itself is considered to be a weak carcinogen.

At first thought the theory is a startling one. It looks as though nature has made a tragic error. How can it be that products of our own bodies' normal functioning—bile acids, neutral sterols, cholesterol—turn against us and make us sick? But nature rarely errs so drastically. The problem lies more with us.

As far as we know, it is possible to live a long and healthy life without ever ingesting food that contains cholesterol. The liver takes care of its own needs for this substance. When we do consume additional cholesterol, greater quantities of bile acids and neutral sterols are synthesized. And there's the rub, as they say. Apparently, normal concentrations of bile acids in the colon are small enough to be relatively harmless. Only larger concentrations, the result of eating food containing high levels of cholesterol, are thought dangerous.

There are also those bacteria to be considered. They are highly desirable tenants of the intestinal tract. We don't want to get rid of them. In fact, we wouldn't be able to live without them. However, people who eat high-fat diets tend to have a somewhat different ratio of various kinds of bacteria in their colons than people who consume relatively little in the way of dietary fat. A high-fat diet seems to favor the growth of what are called "anaerobic bacteria," which are able to live and grow without oxygen. Some researchers believe that these anaerobic bacteria have something to do with the cancer process since they appear to react with the contents of the colon in ways that are different from those of other bacteria.

At the very least we know that when volunteers consume a low-fat diet, as opposed to the standard American diet, even for relatively short periods of time, they excrete significantly smaller quantities of bile acids and neutral sterols and the percentage of anaerobic bacteria in their feces is reduced.

Although the search is still going on, specific carcinogens associated with colon cancer (other than cholesterol and its breakdown products) have not yet been identified. No one yet discounts the possibility that bile salts and neutral sterols work in concert with some more potent carcinogen—perhaps one taken in with our food. But for now we're left with the theory that the colon simply cannot tolerate the presence of bile salts and neutral sterols at slightly elevated levels over a period of years. That in itself may be sufficient to start the cancer process.

It's an unsettling thought. But it's no more farfetched than the now well-accepted concept of a connection between high levels of cholesterol and heart disease.

Interestingly, though populations with a high incidence of heart disease also report a high incidence of colon cancer, the two diseases rarely occur in the same person. Obviously this is to our great good fortune, but it's a puzzle. In an attempt to explain it, some researchers have speculated that there may be individual differences in the way cholesterol is metabolized (made use of) by the body. In one person, for example, cholesterol and other fats may circulate in the blood; the ultimate result is fatty deposits in the arteries (atherosclerosis). In another person, cholesterol may take another metabolic pathway and instead of being retained in the bloodstream be routed to the liver, where it's converted into bile acids and sterols that in turn find their way to the colon. This second person would have lower levels of serum cholesterol (cholesterol in the blood) and a lower risk of coronary artery disease than the first person, even though both might consume identical amounts of dietary cholesterol, but he may run a higher risk of colon cancer. Indeed, colon cancer patients generally don't have the high serum cholesterol readings that are found in heart patients.

It appears that our bodies are not equipped to handle all the cholesterol we may want to put into them. Remember, we don't really *need* any cholesterol, and it's highly probable that when we start eating less of it our health, as a nation and as individuals, will be a whole lot better. One heart specialist, Dr. William E. Connor of the University of Iowa, has stated that if everyone kept his serum cholesterol levels under 190, no one would ever die of atherosclerotic disease. To my knowledge, no cancer specialist has yet made such a positive statement about the effects of eating less cholesterol on the colon cancer rate, but that's not going to stop me from limiting my own cholesterol consumption. What about you?

7

Fiber: What It Can Do for You—and What It Can't

A couple of years ago, Dr. David Reuben, author of *Everything You Always Wanted to Know about Sex* and *Any Woman Can,* wrote another book. It was called *The Save Your Life Diet.* The book became a best seller. Perhaps you read about it. Perhaps you even bought it. In case you didn't, *The Save Your Life Diet* can be summed up in just two words: eat bran.

That's good advice. Most of us *would* be better off if we ate more bran. Or more of anything that is high in fiber. Sometimes called "roughage" or "bulk," fiber is the indigestible residue left over after food has been chemically and physically processed through the body. The skin and stringy "veins" of fruits and vegetables are fiber. Husks, hulls, seeds, in fact all of a plant's "structural" material is fibrous. Fiber adds very little in the way of nutrition but much in the way of volume to the diet. Most Americans don't eat enough of it. If the standard American diet is deficient in anything, it's fiber.

So, like Dr. Reuben, I suggest that you eat more bran and other high-fiber foods. But I'm also going to try to put bran into proper perspective. It's a valuable food but not a miracle food. It's good for us in many ways but it doesn't live up to some of the more extravagant claims made for it.

How did the big bran boom get started in the first place? Well, it all goes back to 1970 when Dr. Denis Burkitt, an Englishman, returned from Africa. There he was struck, among other things, by the fact that Africans who ate the traditional native foods were relatively free of diseases of the gastrointestinal tract—that long, curved and folded system of organs that begins with the stomach, includes the small intestine and large intestine (or colon) and ends at the anus. Black Africans practically never succumb to cancer of the colon. Appendicitis, diverticulosis and hemorrhoids are almost unknown among them. And even heart disease is rare! The same diseases are a scourge to western civilization.

Dr. Burkitt knew that African blacks who migrate to the United States and Britain eventually become just as vulnerable to gastro-intestinal disease—heart disease, too—as native-born Americans and Britons. Therefore, he felt that there must be some environ-mental basis for the Africans' relative immunity to these ailments. Casting about for a logical hypothesis, he settled on diet as the single most reasonable environmental factor to explain what was till then a rather mysterious state of affairs.

Rural black Africans are, in effect, vegetarians. Their diet is mainly one of high-fiber fruits, vegetables and cereal grains. Much of their protein comes from beans and nuts. But a higher fiber content isn't the only difference between the African diet and what most Americans are accustomed to eating. It may not even be the most important difference. You see, the rural African also con-sumes far less fat than the typical American.

Dr. Burkitt was aware of this other difference. He was also aware that the kind of fiber consumed by the Africans is not the kind that is easily available to us in the West. Even so, he was convinced that by eating more of any high-fiber foods we could protect ourselves from certain diseases just as the Africans had.

Dr. Reuben and many others were impressed with Burkitt's African findings. Reuben eventually worked out a diet based on some of them. Bran, the most readily available high-fiber foodstuff in this country, became the key ingredient of the diet, the hinge upon which the whole thing turns.

Eat bran, he says, and protect yourself from cancer of the colon and rectum, heart disease, diverticulosis, varicose veins, appendicitis, hemorrhoids and phlebitis. Obesity is thrown in for good measure.

I applaud the way Dr. Reuben has managed to make millions of Americans more aware of the importance of fiber in the diet. I only wish he'd put in a few good words about the even greater benefits of eating less fat. Ideally we should decrease our fat consumption and increase our fiber consumption *at the same time.* We now know that fiber alone won't accomplish all the wonderful things we had hoped it would.

Let's take a look at fiber and its relationship to colon cancer. In the preceding chapter, on cholesterol, I pointed out that the presence of certain anaerobic bacteria in the colon is thought to have something to do with the disease. More specifically, it is believed that these particular bacteria react with bile acids in the colon, thereby changing them into carcinogenic substances. Work done by Dr. Michael J. Hill of London indicates that there are greater than normal concentrations of anaerobic bacteria in the feces of colon cancer patients and of people who are vulnerable to the disease.

Since populations who eat a high-fat, low-fiber diet have a relatively high rate of colon cancer, some researchers concluded that a greater concentration of anaerobic bacteria in the colon and feces is the *result* of a low fiber–diet. They believed that eating more fiber would change the ratio of anaerobic to aerobic bacteria to a more favorable one. Thus, less of the carcinogen responsible for colon cancer would be produced.

This is an interesting hypothesis, but it's not accepted by everyone. Other scientists, Dr. Sidney Finegold of the University of California, and Dr. W. E. C. Moore and Dr. L. V. Holderman of the Anaerobic Laboratory at Virginia Polytechnic Institute among them, have been unable to confirm it. (These doctors do acknowledge that the fecal bacteria are so various and numerous that differences are hard to detect and evaluate.)

Fiber enthusiasts also claim that the additional bulk it adds to the diet protects against colon cancer because it hastens the elimination process. The theory goes that the less time the fecal stream and its possibly carcinogenic contents remain in contact with the colon, the smaller the risk of colon cancer. The theory doesn't hold up. Rapid "bowel transit," as it's called, may be desirable for any number of reasons, but it doesn't lessen one's chances of developing the disease. The relationship between constipation and colon cancer has been studied time and again and no correlation has been found. In light of what we know now, the person who has one or two bowel movements a week is no more vulnerable to the disease than the person who has daily or twice-daily bowel movements.

The most intriguing claim made for the high-fiber diet is that it lowers serum cholesterol levels. A high level of cholesterol in the blood is *not* a risk factor for cancer of the colon, but it *is* for heart disease. However, the claim that it doesn't matter how much cholesterol we take in with our food as long as we make sure to eat plenty of fiber is dangerous in terms of either disease—and many, many others as well. The truth is, bulk doesn't offset the potentially harmful effects of a diet that is high in cholesterol.

To understand why, let's take another look at some of the information in the chapter on cholesterol. If you remember, bile acids are breakdown products of cholesterol. The liver secretes bile acids into the small intestine where they emulsify fatty substances in the partially digested food. After that, all but about 5 percent of the bile acids are reabsorbed from the small intestine and eventually make their way back to the liver where they are used again in the resynthesis of more bile.

Dr. Reuben and others believe that bulk in the diet "binds" these bile acids, interfering with their reabsorption by the small intestine and thereby reducing the amount of cholesterol resynthesized in the liver. In his book he cites several studies that seem to confirm the hypothesis. However, many other studies don't.

The British medical publication *Lancet* printed in its February 14, 1976, issue an article by A. S. Truswell and Ruth M. Kay of the Nutrition Department of Queen Elizabeth Hospital in London. The article summarized ten separate studies in which the goal was to evaluate bran and its potential for lowering serum cholesterol levels. In all, 135 volunteers were involved. Each consumed anywhere from fourteen to fifty-seven grams of bran daily over periods of time ranging from three to nineteen weeks. Only one group showed a reduction in cholesterol levels.

In November, 1976, Dr. Thomas L. Raymond and his coworkers

at the University of Oregon Health Sciences Center reported that adding fiber to the diets of twelve adult volunteers produced no change in cholesterol levels. Dr. Raymond, speaking at a meeting of the American Heart Association, explained that six of his volunteers had been put on a very low cholesterol diet. Their cholesterol levels went down. But the addition of fiber produced no further lowering. Six other volunteers, put on a high-cholesterol diet, showed high levels of serum cholesterol. No improvement was shown when fiber was added to their diet.

"The message," Dr. Raymond said, "is that fiber alone will not protect you against the effects of a high-cholesterol diet. If you eat the equivalent of four eggs a day and add bran to your diet, the fiber will not help to lower your cholesterol level."

In all of the studies done so far, no fiber tested was as effective in binding bile acids and lowering cholesterol levels as the drugs cholestyramine and cholestipol, which are sometimes administered to patients with very high blood cholesterol levels. Of all the non-drug binding agents, alfalfa fiber does the best job—much better than bran. But even alfalfa fiber was only about one-fifth as effective as the drugs.

If fiber has no effect on the bacterial population of the colon, if its effect on bowel transit time is unimportant with regard to cancer of the colon, if it doesn't lower cholesterol levels, then why should we make an effort to eat more of the stuff?

One reason has to do with the sheer *numbers* of bacteria in the colon and the fecal stream. There are about four billion bacteria per gram dry weight of fecal material. Fully 40 percent of the fecal mass *is* bacteria. Though a high-fiber diet might not alter the ratio of anaerobic to aerobic bacteria in the colon, additional bulk might result in other changes.

For one thing, a large amount of fiber in the fecal stream would dilute the concentration of bacteria. There would be more fiber and fewer bacteria per cubic centimeter. This situation could result in the production of less of the carcinogen that may be involved in colon cancer.

Also, when fecal *volume* is increased, as it is when fiber is added to the diet, the colon walls must expand. When they do, less of the colon's surface area comes into contact with the fecal stream and any carcinogenic substances that might be contained within it.

Stepping up your fiber intake could protect you against diverticulitis, an infectious disease of the colon resulting from inflammation of the diverticula. Diverticula are little "pockets" that are caused by stress or pressure along the weaker portions of the colon wall. These pockets are not "normal," but most Americans have them anyway. In fact, diverticula have been found in about 75 percent of the population over the age of 50. Yet the condition is rare in certain parts of the world. I once worked with a resident physician from the Philippines who told me he had *never* seen diverticula until he came to this country.

Diverticula are hardly ever seen in rural black Africans. Dr. Burkitt, aware of this, believed that their high-fiber diet protected them against the condition. He is undoubtedly right.

As I pointed out a few paragraphs back, more bulk in the diet would increase the volume of the fecal stream, which in turn would cause the colon's walls to expand. With that increase in diameter, there is less lateral pressure on the colon. Under these circumstances, diverticula do not form.

Diverticulitis and a noninfectious version of the same disorder called diverticulosis may indeed be prevented by a high-fiber diet. This kind of preventive medicine can benefit your pocketbook as well as your health. If you ever do experience an attack of diverticulitis, you may be amazed at the sudden concern shown by your insurance company—a concern expressed in the higher premiums you will be asked to pay on any policy purchased after your bout with the illness.

There are more reasons why a high-fiber diet is good for you. Eating more bulk may protect you from a number of other disorders such as appendicitis, anal fissures and hemorrhoids. Fiber's preventive role is somewhat different for each of these diseases. But it always comes down to basically the same thing: a high-fiber diet is what our bodies have adapted to over thousands and thousands of years of evolution. Thus, in many subtle and not so subtle ways, a lack of bulk throws our systems out of whack. Adding more bulk tends to get things back to normal.

But this is a book about diet and cancer and my main reason for suggesting that you eat more fiber has to do with preventing that disease: the more you fill up on bulky, fibrous foods, the easier it will be to cut back on fatty, high-cholesterol foods. (You'll have less room for them!) You see, what the high-fiber people often forget to point out is that the incidence of colon cancer—heart disease, too—correlates better with a diet high in fat than with a diet low in fiber.

Let's also not forget that that additional fiber will dilute the concentration of bacteria in the colon and at the same time cause the colon's walls to expand, thus lessening the effects of carcinogenic substances on that organ.

How can you go about getting more fiber in your diet?

Well, you could do as Dr. Reuben suggests and have a couple of tablespoons of bran before each meal. (Wash it down with a glass of water or fruit juice.) You could also sprinkle it on breakfast cereal, use it as an ingredient in pancakes and muffins, add it to meatloaf or hamburgers and stir it into soups, sauces and gravies. Bran is inexpensive and a good source of bulk. It's available at many supermarkets now, and at almost any health food store.

But you don't need to make a trip to a health food store to get more bulk into your diet. Bran is only one of many foods that are high in fiber. Most fruits and vegetables, provided they're not overcooked, provide bulk. Eat them raw, peel and all, whenever possible. Of course I do not expect you to eat orange peels. Apple peels, however, are quite acceptable. Unfortunately, we do not have a clear-cut definition of how much bulk is needed, nor do we have ideal ways of measuring it. Dr. Reuben, in his book, has implied that 2 ounces of bran is probably enough for anyone in a given day. It is obviously easier to specify portions of bran as a dietary supplement than it is to estimate the amount of fruit and vegetable bulk. I do encourage you to be aware that bulk is necessary and not to discard it from your diet. Some recent studies done with pectin, a derivative of fruit, especially citrus fruit peel, are encouraging. In addition to increasing fecal volume, pectin seems to bind bile products, and initial tests show significant lowering of serum cholesterol. It is difficult to make its taste acceptable, but if this can be corrected pectin will probably be the next "cure-all" health food.

You can also make a number of easy substitutions. Whole grain breads are much higher in fiber than the ordinary white bread made with highly refined flour that so many people have become accustomed to. (I know many people who've switched to whole grain breads and who now find white bread boring, tasteless and devoid of texture. I'm one of them.)

You can also substitute whole grain breakfast cereals for the more refined products. A few to keep in mind are all bran, shredded wheat, 40 percent bran flakes, puffed wheat, oatmeal. Corn flakes, which is an otherwise very good cereal, contains little or no bulk. Rice cereals in general tend to be low in bulk.

As for rice itself, it's worth shopping around for brown rice, which has much more fiber (vitamins, too) than the "polished" white rice. (You may have to go to a health food store to find brown rice.) Wild rice is good, too, but far more expensive.

For more suggestions about how to get additional bulk into your diet, plus a listing of high-fiber foods, see the meal-planning section beginning on page 191.

8

What to Do about Red Meat: Beef, Pork, Lamb and Veal

If the last few chapters have left you with the impression that the Anti-Cancer Diet includes less red meat than you're accustomed to, you've been reading me correctly. Because of its fat and cholesterol content, red meat, our longtime protein mainstay, the entrée around which the rest of a meal is planned, the dieter's delight, the most expensive item in our food budget, the king of foods as it were, has a reduced role in our Anti-Cancer scheme of things.

If you're an "average" American, you've been eating about 58 ounces of red meat each week. That adds up to about 189 pounds a year, an amount that may be equal to (or even exceed) your own body weight.

I'm going to suggest you cut back to six four-ounce servings of *lean* beef, pork, lamb or veal a week. That's twenty-four ounces a week, eighty pounds a year—still a lot more meat than people in many other countries get and more than enough to keep you in excellent health provided you adjust the rest of your diet accordingly.

Of course you know by now that meat is not carcinogenic. No food or type of food that we know of actually *causes* cancer. Part of the trouble with red meat is that it's animal protein. As such, too much of it may "desensitize" the body's immune system, which must stay alert and on the lookout for alien cell structures if it is going to seek out and destroy early clusters of abnormal cells that may be the precursors of cancer. (This is speculation and probably not as important as what follows.)

What really concerns me is the fat content of red meat. As we've seen, the cancers of affluent nutrition correlate very closely with high levels of fat in the diet. Where there is meat you will also find fat. In fact, meat contributes about 42 percent of the total fat content of the average American's diet. Thus, even if you made no other changes in your eating habits, you'd be in a far more favorable position in terms of cancer risk if you simply ate less meat.

The fat content of the various types of red meat depends on the species and the cut, whether it's brisket or short ribs or tenderloin in beef, chops or ham in pork and so on. In the case of beef, the grade is also important. In general "prime" contains more fat than "choice," which is higher in fat than "good." (There are other grades but you're not likely to find them at your local butcher shop or supermarket meat counter.) As a general rule, pork—although differences may be smaller than you suspect—has the highest fat content, followed by lamb, then beef, then veal. Be guided accordingly. And remember, no matter what kind of meat is set before you, trim it of every bit of visible fat before eating.

The degree of doneness of meat also affects its fat content. For example, fat accounts for about 40 percent of the calories in the average steak before cooking. When broiled or pan-fried to the rare stage, that figure is reduced to 28 percent. At medium, 24 percent of the steak's calories are fat and at well done, only 16 percent. These are dramatic and little-known differences. Obviously, we'd all gain by learning to like our meat well done, that is, with as much fat as possible cooked out of it.

When cattle are grass fed rather than grain fed, the fat content of the meat is reduced. Grass isn't converted as efficiently into fat as the corn on which most beef cattle are raised.

Having eaten grass fed beef, I can testify to its quality of taste and texture. It is somewhat more flavorful and less tender than corn fed beef. Argentinians, who are big beef eaters, have a lower rate of those cancers of overnourishment that we've been so concerned with, and most of their beef is grass fed. Whether there is any relationship between their leaner beef and lower cancer rate is open to question. Clearly, though, we aren't necessarily stuck with the beef we have. It is at least theoretically possible to breed and raise cattle and other livestock with all the meaty taste and texture we crave and less of the fat that is so harmful to our health.

By using less meat and only lean meat, you'll also be getting less cholesterol. A high cholesterol intake, as you know, is associated with heart disease and, by other mechanisms, with colon cancer. The American Heart Association firmly states that we could all look forward to better heart health if we kept our cholesterol intake to three hundred milligrams or less per day.

Some cancer specialists have suggested that we halve that figure, slashing cholesterol consumption to 150 milligrams per day or less. This would require a good bit of doing if one were not to become a vegetarian, since almost all food of animal origin contains *some* cholesterol. However, it's entirely possible. As far as we know it's also perfectly safe. The body manufactures all the cholesterol it needs in order to function well and at least one important cancer expert (Dr. Wynder of the American Health Foundation) feels that *any* cholesterol we take in with our food is unnecessary and by definition too much.

My own recommendation is that we aim for the more modest three hundred milligrams a day. The average cut of beef, well cooked and reasonably trimmed of fat, contains about twenty-five milligrams of cholesterol per ounce. There are thirty milligrams of cholesterol in an ounce of pork; twenty-seven in an ounce of lamb; and twenty-six in an ounce of veal. Six four-ounce servings a week of any of these allows you plenty of leeway in selecting other foods. (Slightly different figures are cited by some authorities, depending on the meat sample and how well it was trimmed.)

9

What to Do about Poultry

It used to be that poultry was for festive occasions. Turkey, goose and duck still are, but most of us now view chicken as ordinary everyday fare. And a good thing that is. We'd all be better off if we ate more of this bird, especially if at the same time we reduced red meat intake even further. Chicken is every bit as nutritious as red meat, supplies the same high-quality protein, but contains only half the fat. The same goes for turkey. So I'm decidedly *for* the birds. I'm going to urge you to think chicken and turkey and to substitute either of them for beef, pork, lamb or veal as often as possible.

Contrary to popular opinion, there is no difference in the nutritive value of white and dark meat chicken (or other poultry) except that the white meat contains slightly less fat and somewhat more nicotinic acid. It also has less connective tissue, which makes it a bit easier to digest.

Keep in mind when shopping for chicken that the younger broilers and fryers are less fatty than the older roasting hens and stewing birds.

The general rule that the more well done the less fatty the meat applies to poultry, too. But no matter how done it may be, chicken that is dipped in batter and then deep-fried has no place on the

Anti-Cancer Diet—not unless you carefully remove all the skin before eating it. In fact, skinning a chicken or other fowl before eating is always a good idea, since most of the fat on these birds is in and just under the skin.

Goose and duck have a slightly higher fat content than chicken and turkey. Fat contributes 12 percent of the calories in an ounce of roast goose or duck. Both are comparable in fat content to some cuts of very lean red meat.

As for cholesterol, chicken and turkey both contain about twenty-two milligrams per ounce, which is a modest improvement over beef, at about twenty-five milligrams per ounce.

10

What to Do about Fish
and Other Seafood

Of all foods of animal origin fish is best for reducing your cancer risk. It has several things going for it. For one, no epidemiological study yet has shown a correlation between cancer and a high intake of fresh fish or other seafood. (There does seem to be a connection between eating large amounts of *smoked, pickled, and salted* fish, as is customary in Japan and Iceland, and a high incidence of stomach cancer.)

Aside from that, fish is relatively low in calories per serving. It's also quite low in fat. Depending on the species and the time of year it was caught, fish have a fat content that ranges from about 1 percent to 20 percent. The least fatty fish are the nonoily white-fleshed varieties such as cod, halibut, tuna, shrimp, scallops and perch. Higher (but still very reasonable) amounts of fat are found in salmon, sardine, mackerel, flounder and shad.

The average fish—let's use halibut as an example—contains 2.7 grams of fat per ounce, of which only ½ gram is saturated fat. As you know, in the Anti-Cancer Diet we make very little distinction between saturated and unsaturated fats. Both are undesirable and to be avoided whenever possible. However, a high ratio of unsaturated to saturated fats tends to have an overall cholesterol-lowering effect. That, plus the fact that fish is relatively low in cholesterol to begin with—our average fish (halibut) contains approximately ten milligrams of cholesterol per ounce—makes it a high-quality protein food minus one of the major health drawbacks of other foods of animal origin.

My recommendation is that you include fish on your menu at least once a week, more often if possible. The well-known "Prudent Diet" developed by the New York City Department of Health calls for fish five times a week.

So far we've been talking about the "finny" fish. Shellfish—shrimp, lobster, crab, clams, oysters, et cetera—are another matter. Though their overall fat content is in general very low, they are said to contain rather high levels of cholesterol. In fact, shellfish are taboo in most low-cholesterol diets.

Cholesterol, however, is only one of a number of fat-soluble compounds belonging to the "sterol" family. There is still some question as to whether all of the sterols in shellfish are indeed cholesterol. In fact, some biochemists insist that most shellfish sterols are not cholesterol but related substances.

In any event, the small amount of fat in shellfish is more *un*saturated than saturated, which we know tends to lower cholesterol levels. Thus, an occasional lobster, scallop or shrimp dinner is not necessarily out of place on the Anti-Cancer Diet. Shellfish prices being what they are, not too many of us will want to splurge very often anyway. I know I don't.

11

What to Do about Eggs

The average hen's egg weighs approximately fifty grams, of which 13 percent is protein and 12 percent fat. The yolk contains half of the protein and all of the fat—plus an astounding 253 milligrams of cholesterol. And that is the trouble with eggs.

The egg producers—not the hens, the people in the egg business—contend that eating eggs does not increase the risk of heart disease. But the American Heart Association believes otherwise. It urges us all to keep cholesterol intake down to three hundred milligrams per day and with that restriction it's hard to work in many eggs.

As a result, the egg business is hurting. In 1945, when meat was rationed because of the war, Americans made up for it by eating 400 eggs per person per year. Now we're down to 275 eggs per year and this includes eggs as a "hidden" ingredient in homemade and commercially prepared baked goods and other foods. Interestingly, the heart attack rate (so high in American males) started to turn downward in 1969 and is continuing to show some improvement.

Now that we have evidence that cholesterol is a factor in colon cancer, there is all the more reason to avoid eggs. I personally eat *no* visible eggs—eggs that are scrambled, poached, sunny-side up or otherwise identifiable on my plate. I also stay away from foods that contain eggs as a major ingredient, such as egg noodles and certain pastries. Many of my colleagues do the same.

I must admit I like eggs, but their cholesterol content is just too high to make them acceptable.

Eggs are a variable on the Anti-Cancer Diet. The important goal is to keep cholesterol levels down. People who don't care that much for eggs might as well eliminate them entirely. Egg addicts can allow themselves an egg for breakfast once in a while—but that means going vegetarian for the rest of the day in order to keep cholesterol under the three hundred milligram limit.

An alternative might be to use egg substitutes. These are not artificial eggs at all, but real eggs, modified. Most egg substitutes are made of egg whites and egg yolks from which the cholesterol has been separated by chemical means. In some brands vitamins and minerals are added so that the final product is nutritionally similar to an egg in its original state. My wife and I use egg substitutes in cooking; occasionally we scramble them and use them as the basis for an omelet at breakfast. You might want to do the same. But for poached or sunny-side up, you must use the real thing—if you really must.

For good health, the most important role of the egg is to make chickens.

12

What to Do about
Milk, Butter and Cheese

In a recently published text on nutrition, the section on dairy products leads off with the injunction, "Some milk for everyone daily." Then there is a chart listing the number of ounces of milk that should be drunk daily by people of various ages. To reduce your cancer risk, consider this chart way off base.

While nothing in the literature so far indicates that milk drinking per se is a risk factor for the disease, many of us have for a long time questioned the advisability of "milk for everyone."

Not that milk doesn't sound good on paper. A cup of whole milk is 87 percent water, has 160 calories and 9 grams of protein. Casein, the kind of protein we get in milk, contains all the amino acids the body needs for growth and maintenance. That same cup of milk supplies 12 grams of carbohydrate in the form of lactose, an easily digested sugar.

A cup of milk also gives us 288 milligrams of calcium, and this is one of the things nutritionists rave about. Children do need liberal amounts of calcium for good bone and dental development. Grown-ups also need *some* calcium, but as with so many other things, too much is no good. People who engage in intense physical activity resulting in fluid depletion should be wary of drinking large amounts of milk. When the laborer, dancer or athlete—even the weekend athlete—habitually quenches his or her thirst with milk, there is danger of a calcium overload, and kidney stones may result.

But it's not the high calcium content of milk that I and others interested in cancer prevention object to. It's the fat and cholesterol. A cup of whole milk has nine grams of fat, with at least six of those grams saturated fat—not a favorable proportion. In addition, there are sixty-eight milligrams of cholesterol in eight ounces of milk. (A cup of milk and three ounces of steak contain comparable amounts of cholesterol, but the milk has from 10 to 15 percent more fat.)

My recommendations concerning milk then are:

1. Drink *skim* milk only. It has less than 1 percent fat and only 1.8 milligrams cholesterol per cup but all the other nutrients of whole milk.

2. Assuming you're an adult, drink no more than 2 cups of skim milk a day. Don't guzzle it down after vigorous exercise, either. Choose water, fruit juice or diet soda instead.

Those of you with young children should know that nowadays practically all pediatricians believe there is no need for whole milk after the first year of life. (Some even suggest that mothers switch their babies directly from breast milk or infant formula to skim milk at six months of age or less!) The pediatricians are becoming concerned about the connection between cholesterol and heart disease. They have always been preventive medicine oriented. Therefore their recommendations are exactly in line with Anti-Cancer thinking. Remember, we suspect that a high-fat, high-protein diet started in the early years increases the risk of certain cancers later in life.

A few final comments about milk and cancer. Not too long ago there was some mention in the news media that the decreasing incidence of stomach cancer among the Japanese correlated with their increased milk consumption. Not mentioned was the fact that the Japanese also get far more vitamin C and fewer nitrites in their food than before. Both of these factors (we will take them up in greater detail later) are at least as important in the falling incidence of stomach cancer in Japan as greater milk consumption. Probably more so. We've seen that as the traditional low-fat Japanese diet becomes more like our own, as the Japanese' consumption of red meat, eggs and, yes, milk reaches higher levels, so does their rate of cancers of overnourishment.

What to do about butter?

Since I've already urged you to drink skim milk, which is lower in butterfat than whole milk, it shouldn't surprise you that butter has no place on the Anti-Cancer Diet.

One teaspoon of butter has forty calories and four grams of fat. Of this fat, at least two-thirds is saturated, one-third unsaturated. This is the reverse of the ideal situation. In addition, there are twelve—count 'em, twelve—milligrams of cholesterol in that one little teaspoon of butter.

Substituting corn oil margarine for butter nets you the same number of calories. But in making the switch, cholesterol is entirely eliminated. Furthermore, in corn oil margarine the ratio of unsaturated to saturated fats is a much healthier one.

My recommendation about butter is simple: don't eat it. If you must have a yellow spread on your bread, use corn oil margarine. And use it sparingly.

Now what about cheese?

There are so many different kinds of cheese that it's impossible to make general statements except to point out that *most* cheeses contain less water and calcium and more protein, fat and cholesterol per gram than whole milk. The ratio of saturated to unsaturated fat is about the same as in whole milk.

Fat and cholesterol content vary depending on whether a cheese is made primarily with skim milk, whole milk or whole milk and cream. Obviously, the skim milk cheeses are better from an Anti-Cancer point of view.

American cheese, Cheddar cheese, Monterey Jack and brick cheese are made with whole milk. Most mozzarella, Edam, Gouda and cottage cheese are made with skim milk. The labels of many prepackaged cheeses will tell whether they're made from skim or whole milk, but when buying a cheese that's cut to order you have to take the salesperson's word for it.

Don't use cheese too often, though. Since an ounce on the average has thirty-five milligrams of cholesterol (some cheeses have more, others less), it's not a good bet for the Anti-Cancer Diet. Serve cheese only as a meat substitute; the cholesterol and fat content is comparable.

13

The Cancer-Protective
Fruits and Vegetables

You probably already know that fruits and vegetables are "good for you." You probably even know many of the reasons why. But did you know that some of them may be anti-carcinogenic?

As we've seen, for many years now cancer researchers have been hard at work trying to find patterns in the incidence of the disease, attempting to track down correlations between this or that set of circumstances and this or that form of cancer. Reasonable correlations give us leads indicating where best to invest further research time, energy and funds. They help us to construct hypotheses about what causes cancer and how to prevent it. By now just about everything under the sun has come under the scrutiny of the men and women engaged in cancer research. Including fruits and vegetables.

No positive correlation has been found between eating fresh fruits and vegetables and the incidence of any kind of cancer. It is often the reverse: sometimes, where vegetable and fruit consumption is very high, the incidence of many kinds of cancer is quite low. This has led to speculation about whether there might actually be something about eating large amounts of fruits and vegetables that protects against cancer.

Work done by Dr. L. W. Wattenberg at the University of Minnesota indicates that, yes, indeed, there is!

Dr. Wattenberg carried out a series of strictly controlled experiments with laboratory animals. While working with some of the commercially prepared diets for these animals, he discovered that rats fed with one of them (Purina Rat Chow) seemed to be more resistant to chemical carcinogens than rats fed other diets. He was even able to isolate the key ingredient (even rat chow is a complex of different ingredients). It turned out to be alfalfa meal.

Briefly, and in greatly simplified terms, the alfalfa meal caused an increase in a particular kind of enzyme activity in the rats that tended to detoxify—render harmless—carcinogenic substances administered to the animals.

Lest you begin to worry about whether I'm going to recommend that you supplement your diet with Purina Rat Chow or alfalfa meal, let me assure you, I'm not.

In further testing Dr. Wattenberg found that some other vegetables—the kind people eat—are also capable of stimulating the same kind of increased enzyme activity in the rats as alfalfa meal. The best results were obtained when the animals were fed vegetables of the Brassicaceae family. These are also called cruciferous vegetables, and the family includes Brussels sprouts, broccoli, cauliflower, cabbage and turnips. Similar enzyme activity was also evident when the animals ate large amounts of spinach, celery, lettuce and dill.

The big question is whether these vegetables induce the same cancer-preventive enzyme activity in human beings. We don't yet know for sure, and it may be a while before we do. For obvious reasons we can't take a group of human subjects, feed them lots of broccoli and cauliflower, then expose them to carcinogens in the hope that the vegetables will protect them. But as I mentioned before, we do know that in some populations where vegetable consumption is high and protein intake is adequate the rate of certain kinds of cancer is low.

That's why I believe that we don't need to wait until the results of further testing indicate without doubt that these vegetables inhibit the development of cancer in human beings. Eating more cruciferous vegetables—and other kinds, as well—places us in one of life's rare win-win situations: if they do turn out to be cancer-protective to people, as we suspect they might, we come out ahead; even if they don't induce the same kind of tumor-inhibiting enzyme activity in human beings as they do in test animals, we're still winners. Vegetables and fruits are loaded with vitamins and other essential nutrients; at the same time, most of them are extremely low in fat and calories. In other words, they give us a lot of the good things and practically none of the bad things.

For example, in the United States we get less than 1 percent of our daily ingested fat from fruits and vegetables and only about 10 percent of our calories. But 95 percent of our vitamin C, at least 50 percent of our vitamin A and 25 to 33 percent of our vitamin B_6, thiamine, niacin, magnesium and iron come from this source.

By and large, we probably do not eat enough fresh fruits and vegetables. The all-time high for fruit and vegetable consumption in this country occurred during the postwar years, between 1945 and 1950, probably because meat was still scarce at that time and Americans had to fill up on other things. Then there began a tapering off period when people began to eat less and less fruits and vegetables and more and more fat and animal protein. Government statistics document the shift, but you don't have to go to the bother of looking them up to see how far out of favor fruits and vegetables have fallen. The appearance in the supermarkets of those "he-man meat and potatoes" frozen dinners—for which the big selling point was the *absence* of a vegetable—just about says it all.

By the mid-1970s Americans had once again begun to increase their intake of fruits and vegetables. This could be due to reluctance to pay the suddenly skyrocketing meat prices of the early 70s. (Whenever meat is unavailable or too dear, there is a tendency to try to "make do" with more vegetables.) In any event, the Department of Agriculture reports another upswing in the consumption of fruits and vegetables. Aside from the effect this increase may have on future cancer rates, eating more vegetables means getting more essential nutrients from natural sources.

Take vitamin C, for example. I've suggested elsewhere that you include with each meal a food rich in this vitamin. For most people the mention of vitamin C brings to mind oranges or orange juice. Both are good sources, but there is a wide variety of others that are better or almost as good. They are, in order according to their concentration of this vitamin:

green peppers
broccoli
Brussels sprouts
cauliflower
strawberries
spinach
oranges
cabbage
grapefruit
cantaloupe

Notice how often the cruciferous and other cancer-protective vegetables appear on the foregoing list, and on the ones that follow.

A top-ten list of fruits and vegetables high in vitamin A includes:

carrots
sweet potatoes
spinach
cantaloupe
apricots
broccoli
peaches
cherries
tomatoes
asparagus

(For some reason, people have been eating fewer and fewer sweet potatoes of late. This is unfortunate, because they're such good sources of vitamin A.)

The fruits and vegetables that are richest in niacin, an important B-complex vitamin, are:

peas
corn
potatoes
asparagus

lima beans
peaches
artichokes
broccoli
Brussels sprouts

Riboflavin, another one of the B-complex vitamins, is most abundant in the following:

broccoli
spinach
asparagus
Brussels sprouts
peas
corn
lima beans
snap beans
cauliflower
green peppers

Thiamine, still another B-complex vitamin, is found in highest concentrations in the following:

peas
lima beans
asparagus
corn
cauliflower
potatoes
watermelon
sweet potatoes
spinach
broccoli
Brussels sprouts

Of all the trace elements, iron is the one we're most concerned about from an Anti-Cancer point of view. Old Popeye was right; spinach does have the highest concentration of this all-important mineral. It is followed by:

lima beans
peas
Brussels sprouts
artichokes
broccoli
cauliflower
strawberries
asparagus
snap beans

The richest vegetable and fruit sources of calcium are:

broccoli
spinach
snap beans
lima beans
artichokes
cabbage
tangerines
celery
carrots
Brussels sprouts

Potassium, another important trace element, is most abundant in:

lima beans
watermelon
spinach
artichokes
potatoes
Brussels sprouts
broccoli
bananas
carrots
celery

To sum up, an overall ranking of fruits and vegetables according to their value in human nutrition would put broccoli in first place. The other gold medal winners would be, in order:

spinach
Brussels sprouts
lima beans
peas
asparagus
artichokes
cauliflower
sweet potatoes
carrots

Once again, I want to call your attention to the fact that the vegetables that are, we hope, cancer-protective turn up over and over again on all of these lists. I doubt that this is a coincidence.

The best nutritional value is always found in the *freshest* fruits and vegetables. What happens to them between the time they're harvested and the time they finally appear on the table to be eaten is extremely important. Improper storage decreases nutritional value; so does allowing too long a time to elapse before eating.

You should also know that unless produce is promptly refrigerated—or better still, *eaten*—the harmless and naturally occurring nitrates they contain may be converted by bacteria into nitrites in much the same way as they are in processed meats. In fact, naturally occurring nitrates in vegetables can—if the produce remains unrefrigerated—result in a nitrite content as high as that of some processed meats. So proper storage (or quick eating) of just purchased vegetables is as important if not more important as the precautions I will suggest about nitrites in processed meats in chapter 16.

Proper storage is somewhat tricky because not all produce benefits by the same degree of coldness. For instance, potatoes stored at thirty-two degrees Fahrenheit lose more vitamin C than if stored at fifty or even sixty degrees. Asparagus left at room temperature loses most of its B-complex vitamins within three days; stored on crushed ice for as long as two weeks, it not only retains but actually shows some gain in these vitamins.

Storage techniques are important to everyone, even people who grow their own fruits and vegetables, since produce cannot stay on the tree or in the ground indefinitely. For this reason I'm including Table 1, which indicates the best temperatures for storing many of the more common fruits and vegetables. Since most of us have only one refrigerator, it is impossible to duplicate some of these ideal storage temperatures in the home. This is not necessarily a problem. It only means that you should serve and eat very soon after purchasing those fruits and vegetables that are quickly perishable under "ordinary" (that is, standard home) refrigeration.

1.   DESIRABLE STORAGE TEMPERATURES

Product	Temperature (°F)
Apples	32–40
Avocados	
Most varieties	45
West Indian varieties	55
Bananas (green)	56–60
Cherries (sweet)	32
Cranberries	36–40
Dates	40–50
Grapefruit	50–60
Limes	48–50
Oranges	
Arizona & California	40–44
Florida & Texas	32–40
Asparagus	32–36
Beans (snap)	45
Cantaloupe	35–40
Celery	32
Cucumbers	45–50
Honeydew melon	45–50
Lettuce	32
Onions (dry)	32–40
Peppers (sweet)	45–50
Potatoes	
Early crop	50–60
Late crop	40–50

You'll find cooking and serving techniques in chapter 25, How to Cook the Anti-Cancer Way.

14

What to Do about Cereals

What nutritionists call "cereals" or "grains" (or "cereal grains") are the starchy edible seeds of grassy plants. Wheat, rice, corn and oats have been a mainstay of the human diet for thousands of years. Not only did they provide nourishment for our ancestors, they also played a big role in "civilizing" them. It wasn't until they discovered that these plants could be easily grown with a minimum expenditure of energy that people stopped their wandering in search of food and settled down in communities to grow it.

The different grains are similar in many respects. They are lacking in calcium and vitamins A (except for corn) and C, but are reasonably good sources of many other nutrients. Some grains are high in protein, but not the kind that we call "complete" protein. They lack one or more of the essential amino acids. However, when grains are supplemented by two or three other foods containing calcium, vitamins A and C and those missing amino acids, the balance becomes a nutritious one, and people all over the world have managed to survive quite well on a grain-based diet.

I'm going to suggest that you make an effort to get more *whole* grains into your diet—partly because they'll add bulk, and partly to make up for the smaller amounts of red meat, eggs and dairy products called for on the Anti-Cancer Diet. Just remember that the two words *whole grains* are important here. Highly refined grain products, as we shall see, add little or no bulk and not very much of anything else but calories.

Populations whose diets are based on grain generally have a low incidence of those forms of cancer that we've been calling the cancers of affluent nutrition. However, in those places where grains are the only foodstuffs available, the people often suffer from nutritional deficiencies of one kind or another that may result in cancers of another kind, those usually associated with malnourishment, such as some cancers of the esophagus and pharynx.

Still another cancer, primary cancer of the liver, is directly traceable to a mold that thrives in grain and nuts that have been improperly stored. Improper storage leads to the production of a contaminant, aflatoxin, which is about as potent a carcinogen as you will find in nature. Liver cancer, which has less than a 5 percent cure rate, is caused by eating aflatoxin-contaminated grain or nuts. The disease is endemic in those very same parts of Africa where Dr. Burkitt found inhabitants relatively free of colon cancer and other diseases of the gastrointestinal tract. We in the United States are fortunate indeed that grain storage and milling procedures are such that aflatoxin contamination is not a problem.

But those same safe storage and milling procedures that protect us from aflatoxin have robbed us of much that is valuable in cereal grains. (In fact, it's been said that no self-respecting fungus or bacterium would go near the refined white flour used in most of our bread and baked goods because it's nutritionally so poor that the organism would starve.) In the interest of a longer "shelf life," the germ and the bran layers—the most nutritious parts of the wheat berry—are often removed. These are the parts that contain fat—very small amounts of fat to be sure, but enough of it to turn the flour rancid under prolonged storage or storage in less than ideal conditions.

Commercial bakeries attempt to make up for the loss of nutrients by putting some of them back in their products—but these added vitamins and minerals are generally the very ones that are readily available from other sources, so the effort and expense seem unjustified. A better solution would be for bakeries either to mill their own flour from whole grain as needed or to purchase freshly milled whole grain flour for each day's use. If they used only very freshly milled whole grain flour, our bread and other commercial baked goods would be nutritionally far better products and at the same time there would be no danger of aflatoxin contamination.

A few commercial bakeries make a point of saying on their labels that their product is "made from stone ground flour," or simply "stone ground." These breads are probably preferable to others because when a stone mill is used, the wheat berry is coarsely ground; as a result, less of its more nutritious parts are separated out than in a regular steel milling process.

Incidentally, if you do much of your own baking and have access to a source of wheat that is still in grain form, you can make your own coarse whole wheat flour, as my wife and I sometimes do. You simply put the grain into a blender, secure the lid and turn the machine on. In a matter of seconds you have your own freshly milled flour, nutritionally intact and ready to be used in almost any recipe that calls for regular flour.

Just to give you an idea of the difference between whole wheat flour and refined cake or pastry flour, here's the nutritional rundown on each:

One hundred grams (about one half cup) of whole wheat flour has 333 calories, 13 grams of protein, less than 1 gram of fat, 71 grams of carbohydrate and 2.3 grams of fiber. It's rich in phosphorus, has moderate amounts of iron, thiamine and riboflavin, but no vitamin A or C.

One hundred grams of white cake flour has 364 calories, 8 grams of protein, 1 gram of fat, 79 grams of carbohydrate and only .2 gram of fiber. It contains less than one-fourth of the phosphorus of whole wheat flour, little or no iron, thiamine or riboflavin, and no vitamin A or C.

Rice is second only to wheat in the quantity grown and used to feed human beings. The polishing process in rice, which makes it easier to store over periods of time, is similar to the milling process in wheat in that it removes much of the nutritional value. As with wheat, the vitamins and minerals that get lost in the polishing process may be added later on.

Rice has fewer calories and considerably less protein (only 2 or 3 percent, in fact) than wheat. There is virtually no fat in rice. Its fiber content depends on how it's been processed, but at best it's quite low. Rice has very little sodium; therefore hypertension is often treated in part by placing the patient on a rice diet. The reducing diet based on rice that was popular a few years back was a good one for taking off pounds, but the person who eats only rice for any extended period of time always ends up with multiple nutritional deficiencies.

Corn was totally unknown outside the Western Hemisphere before the time of Columbus. Now it's grown throughout the world wherever land can be irrigated or where there is more than eight inches of rainfall during the growing season. Corn is a valuable food for human beings, but much of the total annual production in this country goes to fattening livestock.

Corn has slightly more protein than rice, is 1 percent fat and 21 percent carbohydrate. It's relatively low in the B-complex vitamins, but yellow corn is a good source of vitamin A (white corn has only traces of this vitamin).

Corn oil, extracted from the kernel, has more than three times more polyunsaturated than saturated fatty acids. Therefore, it's an important element in diets that are designed to lower serum cholesterol levels.

Cornstarch is pure carbohydrate with no protein or fat, vitamins or minerals. It finds its way to our tables in many forms—in baked goods, salad dressings, packaged mixes; as a thickener, filler, moisture absorbent and "carrier" for fats and flavors. Food technology has advanced to the point where even good old cornstarch can be and often is chemically modified. A recent tv documentary raised questions about the safety of these chemical procedures. No valid scientific study has yet indicated that they present any danger to our health.

Compared to wheat, rice and corn, oats are relatively unimportant in this country's diet. Approximately 1.5 million bushels are produced each year, but nearly 90 percent of it goes to feeding livestock.

Oats, as raw grain, are high in protein and relatively high in fat. They're a good source of vitamin B_1. However, by the time they're processed the protein is down to only 2 percent, the fat to 1 percent, and the thiamine content is considerably reduced. Oats are a fairly good source of vitamin E and provide about as much of the other B-complex vitamins as wheat and rice.

With fruit and maybe some skim milk, oatmeal, with its low fat content, makes a fine breakfast—far superior from an Anti-Cancer point of view to the standard scrambled or sunny-side-up egg(s) and bacon.

Other cereal grains are the sorghums, which are used in making molasses and some sugars, and rye, used in making bread and occasionally other baked goods. The sorghums are nutritionally similar to corn, while rye is closer to wheat but has somewhat less protein.

15

How to Get Alternative Protein

Meat and other animal products have always been our primary sources of protein in the United States and other rich western countries. No one expects it to be otherwise—not for a long time at any rate. However, the days of cheap meat seem to be past. We may never know them again. The cost of dairy products is on the rise as well, and even fish is no longer the bargain it once was.

Cost aside, animal products tend to be high in fat, especially saturated fat and cholesterol. As we've seen, the affluent diet, high in fat and cholesterol, is a risk factor in various types of cancer (not to mention stroke, heart disease and other ailments). There is also the theory—not yet proved but promising enough to take into consideration—that an oversupply of animal fats and protein tends to confuse the body's immune system, making it less able to seek out and destroy the small early clusters of cancer cells that are believed to be formed in the body every day.

All of this taken together leads inescapably to the thought that substituting nonanimal protein for animal protein—at least occasionally—might be a very good idea indeed.

Nutritionists have long considered animal protein to be superior to plant protein because it is "complete," which means all of the various amino acids necessary to good health are present in it.

Plant protein is different. It's protein, all right, but no matter what kind of plant it comes from, it will be lacking in one or more of those amino acids.

Soybeans and other legumes, peas and beans for example, are high in protein—but it is protein deficient in the amino acid methionine.

Many of the cereal grains—wheat, corn, rice and the rest—contain fair amounts of protein but are lacking in one or more amino acids. (Wheat is low in lysine, corn and rice are low in tryptophan.)

But—and here's the important part—soybeans and the other legumes contain the amino acids that are missing from the cereal grains, while the cereal grains have plenty of methionine, which is absent from the legumes. So though the proteins from either legumes or cereal grains are incomplete, they're incomplete in different ways. If you combine a legume and a cereal grain you get complete protein!

(It's fascinating, I think, that long before anyone knew anything about amino acids, long before there were scientists in fact, the peasant populations of various parts of the world were eating cheap, complete protein combinations of legumes and cereal grains. Think of the corn and beans of the American Indian, the Oriental rice and soybean dishes, the lentils and wheat of the Middle East.)

In mentioning legumes and cereal grains as an alternative source of complete protein, I'm not suggesting that you give up meat eating entirely. I personally am not ready to take that step and perhaps I never will be. As I've pointed out before, I don't believe it's necessary to eliminate meat and other animal products in order to protect yourself from cancer and other diseases associated with a high-fat, high-cholesterol diet. But it's clear that we have to make some modifications in that diet. Eating less meat and other animal protein is one change we can make. Eating more vegetable protein is another.

The meal-planning section of this book contains several recipes that combine legumes and grains. (You'll find dozens more in any good vegetarian cookbook.) If you've always been a meat and potatoes type, you may be surprised at how tasty and satisfying some of them are. At least give them a try and—assuming you like them—serve them on a once-in-a-while basis.

No discussion of alternative sources of protein would be complete without a few more words about the lowly soybean, which, as it turns out, isn't so lowly after all. The ancient Chinese designated it, along with rice, wheat, barley and oats, one of the "five sacred grains" (though of course the soybean isn't a grain at all), and it has been important in Oriental nutrition for thousands of years. Yet many westerners act as though the soybean had just been invented.

What *is* new about the soybean is its use as the main ingredient in something called "textured vegetable protein," a versatile high-protein substance that can be sliced, cubed, cut into chunks and formed into rolls and granules. It can also be canned, frozen or dried. It can be eaten pretty much as is, or it can be flavored so that it begins to resemble bacon, beef or chicken in taste. (Textured vegetable protein may also be made from wheat gluten.)

Textured vegetable protein contains no cholesterol, though some animal fat is added to some varieties. Its fat content is generally low but varies according to how it's been processed and is much higher in some types than others. It retains its shape and texture during cooking and can be pan-fried without shrinking, or baked, grilled, stewed or what have you. Pound for pound its cost is much lower than meat, yet its nutritive value in some cases is comparable to animal products. It may very well be the food of the future. It's my guess that this substance will be turning up more and more often as an ingredient in commercially prepared foods and that its use in the home will increase substantially within the next decade or so.

In fact, textured vegetable protein is with us right now. The chicken and beef analogs that I sampled on my visit with the Seventh-day Adventist chaplain and his family were textured vegetable protein. Its use as an "extender" in chili con carne, meatballs, meat loaf, hamburger, et cetera, by the National School Lunch Program is well known (rations of 30 percent soy protein to 70 percent meat are now allowable).

How does this substance rate from an Anti-Cancer point of view? To begin with, soybeans—the major ingredient—are not incriminated in any epidemiological study. The processing techniques that turn soybeans into textured vegetable protein seem to be harmless and apparently do not result in significant chemical contamination. That, plus low cost and the fact that most of us now eat more meat than we need—and more than is good for us—makes it look as though textured vegetable protein could someday have an important place in our diet, either as a food in its own right, or to make "the real thing"—meat—go farther.

16

Nitrates, Nitrites, Nitrosamines: What Are They? And What Can You Do about Them?

Not long ago someone I know took me aside at a party and asked for what we used to call "the lowdown" on nitrates. He said he'd read several items in the paper telling about the dangers of nitrates in food, warning that these substances might cause cancer and were dangerous to human health in other ways as well.

I told him it wasn't nit*rates* but nit*rites* that were the culprits and launched into a quick explanation (I have to admit I'm often reluctant to discuss medicine in off-hours). When I mentioned the word "nitrosamine" he shook his head and held up a hand for me to stop. "Okay, obviously you've got to be a chemist to understand this sort of thing. Let's drop the subject."

My friend is a businessman, a very sharp fellow, someone who tries to be up on what's happening in the world, yet I'm not surprised that the nitrate–nitrite–nitrosamine business was confusing to him. Those newspaper stories and magazine articles pointing out the dangers of nitrites in our food *are* confusing. But what they're trying to tell us is important. In this chapter we're going to clear up some of the confusion and consider a few ways to protect ourselves from nitrites and nitrosamines.

First of all, nitrates and nitrites are two different things. Nitrates are harmless substances that occur almost everywhere but are

especially abundant in certain kinds of soil. They are a major
component of fertilizers, both the man-made inorganic kind and
the organic fertilizers and manure. Plants depend on nitrates as an
important source of nitrogen. In fact, without nitrogen we'd have
no plant life on earth. Some vegetables actually concentrate nitrates within their tissues. Spinach, rhubarb and beets, to name just
three, absorb and store nitrates from the soil in amounts as high as
.1 to .5 percent of their total volume. Even such high levels of
nitrate in vegetables represent no danger to our health so long as
nitrate remains nitrate and is not converted by bacteria into nitrite.

This transformation occurs quite "naturally," however, when
vegetables are improperly transported or stored, or when long
periods elapse between picking and eating. (See chapter 13 on the
importance of proper storage and/or prompt use of vegetables.)
For now let's turn to nitrates used as preservatives. That's where
most of the nitrate controversy is focused.

Nitrates and nitrites are used to prevent spoilage and preserve
the color of such processed meats as ham, bacon, hot dogs, cold
cuts and corned beef. Much of nitrate's effectiveness as a preservative depends on its conversion by bacteria into ni*trite*. Nitrite isn't
all bad. It inhibits the growth of some of the most deadly organisms known, including Clostridium botulinum, the bacterium that
causes the dread and almost always fatal botulism poisoning.
Botulism is very rare in this country nowadays, partly because of
nitrates and nitrites as preservatives and partly because of improved methods of handling, refrigerating, cooking and packaging
processed meat.

But nitrites are extremely active in the chemical sense, which
means that they combine quickly and easily with other compounds.

For example, a condition called methemoglobinemia may occur when nitrites, taken into the body with food or drinking water,
react with the iron carried by hemoglobin in the blood. As a result,
the blood cannot deliver enough oxygen to the various parts of the
body. The victim, almost always a young child (and the younger
and smaller the child, the more pronounced the reaction) suffers
severe oxygen deprivation, becomes short of breath and may turn
blue. Methemoglobinemia is rare. Many busy pediatricians may
never see a case of it. If proper diagnosis is made, treatment is
simple and recovery complete.

The legal limit of nitrite in processed meat products is .02 percent, and it has been estimated that an adult would have to eat at least fifty hot dogs at a sitting, or between three and six pounds of ham or corned beef, for the nitrite level in his or her system to reach the point where methemoglobinemia becomes a possibility. Children's small bodies are of course more vulnerable. Many doctors, health officials and consumer advocates are urging that nitrates and nitrites in baby foods be eliminated entirely or reduced even more drastically than they already have.

People who make their own sausages at home have been known to add too much of the white, powdery crystalline sodium nitrite to the meat mixture, and there has been at least one death reported as the result of mistaking sodium nitrite for garlic powder. In short, nitrite is a substance to be wary of.

But it is not methemoglobinemia or the hazards of accidental overuse with which all those recent newspaper and magazine articles are most concerned. The big to-do has to do with the relationship of nitrites to cancer. Here, somewhat simplified, is how the chemical and the disease appear to be linked.

As I mentioned, nitrates are added to processed meat to preserve its color and prevent spoilage. Nitrites are formed as the result of bacterial action. (The maximum amount of nitrate that can be legally added to meat is .05 percent, or five hundred parts per million; the nitrite level in the finished products must not exceed .02 percent, or two hundred parts per million.)

So far, no problem. However, if any of another kind of chemical compound called "secondary amines" are present in the stomach when the meat is eaten, the nitrites in the meat may combine with the amines to form still another kind of compound called a "nitrosamine."

Some nitrosamines are highly potent carcinogens. As little as from two to five parts per million of one kind of nitrosamine (dimethylnitrosamine) in the daily diet of rats has resulted in cancer. One-time exposures to larger doses have also produced malignant tumors. Nitrosamines are among the few compounds that appear to cause cancer in all members of the animal kingdom. All animals exposed to them, including monkeys, eventually develop cancer of one kind or another.

Now let's take a closer look at those compounds called secondary amines. Where do they come from? How would they happen to be in our stomachs in the first place?

Unfortunately, there are amines lurking everywhere. They occur in a few of the foods we eat, in some beverages, in tobacco smoke and in many drugs.

When I asked the head pharmacist at my hospital, St. Luke's in Kansas City, about drugs containing amines that might react with nitrites, he indicated with a sweeping motion of his arm that nearly half the compounds in the hospital pharmacy belong in that category. As might be expected because of their name, many antihistamines contain amines. So do many sedatives. The tranquilizers Librium and Valium, two of the most commonly prescribed drugs in the country, have amines in their chemical makeup. (Animals fed high dosages of nitrites and one or the other of the two tranquilizers tended to develop tumors of the central nervous system.) Cold remedies, including the kind sold over the counter, as well as many antibiotics, are compounded partly with members of the amine family of chemicals.

More discouraging still, when our bodies metabolize protein, amino acids—which are also amines—are produced. The presence of amino acids in our bodies is inevitable. In fact, they're essential to health and life itself.

The truth is, it's impossible to avoid amines. And amines combined with nitrites form carcinogenic nitrosamines. That's the bad news.

Now the good news. Working with nitrites and the antibiotic Terramycin, which contains amines, researchers at the Epley Institute for Cancer Research at the University of Nebraska found that the two combined did indeed yield a carcinogenic nitrosamine (dimethylnitrosamine, to be exact). But they also discovered that the reaction could be prevented if a small amount of ascorbic acid—vitamin C—was present.

This discovery led to experiments involving other nitrites and amine compounds. While there was considerable variation in the types of compounds used, the researchers found that in environments similar to the human gastrointestinal tract, most of these nitrite-amine fusions could be prevented when small amounts of ascorbic acid were added.

It was a discovery of enormous interest to cancer researchers and everyone else concerned with preventive medicine. Imagine! Just a little bit of ascorbic aid—vitamin C—cancels out the chemical reaction that results in some of the most potent carcinogens we know of. (On second thought, perhaps the simplicity of it all isn't so amazing. Perhaps our instincts in selecting a well-balanced diet have always led us to an attempt to include some foods that are high in vitamin C with our meals. Still, it's interesting that so many of our favorite combinations should turn out to be so advantageous: the vitamin C in the tomato in the BLT sandwich cancels out the nitrites in the bacon; the vitamin C in the cabbage counteracts the nitrites in the corned beef; and so on.)

It's important to understand that the nitrite-amine reaction can be prevented only if the ascorbic acid is present in the stomach at the same time as the nitrites and amines. In other words, a glass of orange juice or a multivitamin pill first thing in the morning would have little or no effect with regard to the nitrites in the liverwurst sandwich you eat at lunchtime.

For that reason I'm going to suggest that each meal you eat include a food that is rich in vitamin C. (You'll find a listing of these foods on page 89.) Vitamin C is especially important when the bill of fare includes hot dogs, ham, bacon, corned beef, cold cuts or other processed meat products that contain nitrites. (Get into the habit of reading labels; by law, nitrates and nitrites must be listed as ingredients if they are used.)

If for some reason you cannot include some food rich in vitamin C with a meal, it might not be a bad idea to take a vitamin C supplement with the meal. In most instances this seems unnecessary. I am opposed to the large doses of vitamins commonly supplied in most tablets or capsules. I suggest that the with-meal supplement not be greater than 100 mg. in tablet or capsule form.

I'm very much in favor of the first alternative because reasonable selection and mixing of foods should be all that's necessary for good dietary health. Vitamin supplements are all right if you feel more comfortable with them, but at this time there is no generally accepted evidence that additional vitamins reduce cancer risks. The situation may change with the introduction of vitamin A analogs in the future. (More on this later.)

There's more good news concerning the nitrate problem, and it has to do with technological developments in the food industry. To put the news into historical perspective, let's keep in mind that before the advent of refrigeration the *only* way to prevent processed meat from being contaminated by the organisms that cause botulism was to add nitrates. Then, with refrigeration and improved sterilization techniques, the need for nitrates and nitrites began to decrease. Recently it was shown that when meat is kept at temperatures below two degrees Celsius (that's about thirty-five degrees Fahrenheit), nitrate added as a preservative does not convert as readily to nitrite. It's also been shown that at those low temperatures the approximately 150 parts per million of sodium nitrite added to meat (the current rate at which the chemical can be used) dissipate. By the time the meat is eaten, the original 150 parts per million is down to 10.

In other words, with new processing and refrigeration techniques smaller amounts of nitrates and nitrites can deliver as much protection against spoilage and botulism as larger amounts did in the past. Some experts have suggested that with very clean processing plants, quick handling and adequate refrigeration, we'll no longer need nitrates and nitrites as preservatives. Others are not so optimistic.

Whether we ever do arrive at a point where these chemicals can be completely phased out, the fact remains that there has been a declining need for them over the years and a corresponding drop in their use. As a population, we probably get only about one-tenth as much of these compounds in our food as our parents did in the mid-1930s, and as a result we've seen a drop in stomach cancer rates in this country. (We're beginning to see the same kind of tapering off in the incidence of stomach cancer in Japan. This may have to do with the gradual change in Japanese eating habits. Salting has long been a traditional method of food preparation and preservation in Japan, but Japanese crude salt contains very high levels of sodium nitrite. With the shift to western-style foods, less salt and smaller quantities of sodium nitrite are being consumed.)

If meat processors continue to use smaller amounts of nitrates and nitrites (it looks as though they can, and with pressure from the public and the federal government, they will), we should see an even greater drop in the rate of stomach cancer here.

Of course, we have to remember that nitrites play a part in preserving the color of processed meat. With fewer or no nitrites we'll be seeing lots of whitish ham and gray-toned hot dogs around. I for one am ready to accept them. What about you?

17

Deficiencies: Just How Important Are They in the Cancer Process?

For a while scientists did entertain the possibility that all cancer was the result of nutritional deficiencies. But that was years ago. Now we have a better idea of the complexity of the disease. We see that there is no *one* cause, no *one* cure, and no *one* simple preventive measure—nutritional or otherwise—that will guarantee protection from it.

We also know that in this country nutritional *excesses* play a bigger role in the incidence of cancer than a lack of vitamins or other nutrients in our food. (In a way, it's too bad it couldn't be the other way around. If it were, we could simply add the missing substances to our drinking water or to flour or some other universal food and all malignancy would disappear. Now that *would* be cause for rejoicing!)

Still, there are enough bits of evidence to keep researchers interested in the role of certain deficiencies as factors in the development of certain forms of the disease. In this chapter we're going to focus on a few of them.

Let's start out with vitamin A. A good supply of vitamin A is essential to healthy, normal "epithelium"—the cells that make up the skin and the linings of the hollow organs of the digestive system, the respiratory system (including the lungs) and the urinary tract.

Nutritionists and clinicians have seen how a deficiency of vitamin A results in changes in the epithelium of the mouth, the upper respiratory tract and even in the lower urinary tract and cervix. Some of these changes are "premalignant," which means that tumor cells are present but that those cells are relatively harmless and may remain harmless. Yet they may develop into cancer; they are something in between normal and cancerous cells.

Premalignant tissue changes are always cause for concern and researchers have long been investigating the relationships among vitamin A deficiency, premalignant changes in the epithelium and cancer.

Unfortunately most deficiencies are enormously complex. Many epidemiological studies show a high rate of certain kinds of cancer in malnourished populations. But in those areas where one vitamin or other nutritional element is missing from the diet, multiple nutritional deficiencies usually exist as well. It's hard to single out *the* cancer-causing deficiency, to know whether the high rate of cancer is the result of only one deficiency or a spectrum of deficiencies.

A controlled deficiency pattern *can* be produced with laboratory animals. Researchers discovered that animals placed on vitamin A–deficient diets developed more tumors when exposed to carcinogenic chemicals than animals maintained on balanced diets. Those tumors tended to occur in the lung and esophagus. Among human beings, smokers are at high risk for both kinds of tumors.

Then a group of British scientists discovered reduced levels of vitamin A in the blood of virtually all the lung cancer patients they studied.

Put the animal data together with the information gathered in lung cancer studies and the inevitable question arises: Does a vitamin A deficiency—which we already know causes premalignant changes in the epithelium of the throat and lungs of human beings—make people more vulnerable to the carcinogens in tobacco smoke and polluted air?

To answer with an unqualified yes would be jumping the gun, but it certainly does appear that way. However, I'm not going to suggest that smokers and city dwellers who must breathe polluted air take large supplemental doses of vitamin A. For one thing, excesses of vitamin A are toxic to human beings. For another, vitamin A in excess actually *promotes* the growth of tumors in laboratory animals. So vitamin A levels need to be kept in balance, neither falling too low nor climbing too high. Vitamin A in "megadoses" is not the answer.

But vitamin A "retinoids" may be, if important animal data apply to man. Retinoids are a kind of synthetic vitamin A which appear to have all the properties of naturally occurring vitamin A, minus its toxicity at high dose levels. (They are also called vitamin A analogs.) These substances have been shown to promote the growth of healthy, normal tumor-resistant epithelial tissue in test animals and we have no reason to believe they will not do the same in human beings. (Clinical trials with humans are just getting under way.)

Retinoids constitute one of the most exciting recent developments in cancer research. Their implications are truly awesome. They point to a time when, assuming the substances are harmless to human beings, all of us, smokers and nonsmokers alike, will be protected from epithelial cancer, including lung cancer, by a daily dose of vitamin A retinoids! Pie in the sky projects have appeared before, only to crumble with additional study. Hopefully, this promise is for real.

Until that day, my recommendation as to vitamin A has to be simply that you get adequate amounts of it in the food you eat. (Almost all red, orange and yellow fruits and vegetables, and green vegetables such as spinach, broccoli and asparagus are excellent sources.) Or, if you insist, invest in a good multivitamin preparation, one that includes riboflavin (one of the B-complex vitamins) and vitamin C, though in general I feel that vitamins are unnecessary for people who eat properly.

Interestingly, vitamin A—as well as vitamin C and riboflavin— are conspicuously low (one might almost say they're absent) in the diet of many people who live in certain parts of Iran. In those same areas there is a very high incidence of cancer of the esophagus—in some localities twice the incidence in any other part of the world. In other parts of Iran, the rate of cancer of the esophagus is pretty much the same as in most of the rest of the world.

Tobacco and alcohol are used infrequently in that part of the world, and researchers believe that men and women in the high-risk areas are vulnerable to malignancies of the esophagus because of extreme dietary deficiencies. These people live mainly on bread, goat's milk and tea. But researchers also believe that deficiencies alone aren't responsible for the cancer, that the local custom of drinking tea at very hot temperatures—in some cases just below boiling—has a lot to do with it. In other words, the deficiency results in abnormal epithelial changes in the esophagus, while the hot tea provides an additional insult to the tissues. The two conditions set the stage for the development of cancer.

It's a familiar story: a dietary factor (in this case, not enough of certain nutritional elements; though as we've seen, it could also be an excess of certain nutrients) makes the body more vulnerable to an environmental carcinogen or some other cancer-causing substance, and the final outcome is malignancy.

In a few other areas where the incidence of cancer of the esophagus is high—including some parts of Russia and China—the population is in general malnourished. It seems that only in countries like our own, where nutrition is considered adequate, do smoking and alcohol become important in the development of the disease.

An interesting situation exists in Sweden. There, cancer of the esophagus and pharynx (the area just behind the tongue) in males is associated with heavy drinking and smoking. But Swedish women, who rarely smoked or drank until recently, also had a high incidence of the two cancers. Medical researchers were able to identify a disorder called Plummer-Vinson syndrome as a contributing factor to cancers of the esophagus and pharynx in women. Plummer-Vinson syndrome probably starts early in life; it's characterized by anemia and epithelial changes in the pharynx and esophagus. After several years malignant degeneration takes place.

We don't usually think of Sweden as one of the undernourished countries of the world, but in the rural north of that country, where Plummer-Vinson syndrome appears most frequently, the winters are long and fresh vegetables and meat are scarce during the cold months, so that the people suffered some dietary deficiencies. The Swedish government took action in 1944 and ruled that iron and vitamins be added to the flour. Since then Plummer-Vinson syndrome has been appearing less and less frequently and there has been a corresponding drop in the incidence of cancer of the pharynx and esophagus in women. In fact, Swedish women today are at only about half the risk for these two cancers as Swedish men.

Here we have a concrete, documented example of how the cancer rate was reduced as a result of making up for deficiencies—in this case vitamins and iron—in the diet of a population. But why did the correction of a nutritional deficiency make such a great difference in the cancer rate of Swedish women, but not of Swedish men? The best explanation is that the women who later developed Plummer-Vinson syndrome probably were born with a predisposition to the disease which was later offset by supplemental iron and vitamins. Swedish males, it's believed, did not inherit this predisposition, but in middle age became susceptible to cancer of the pharynx and esophagus as a result of heavy drinking and smoking and the same iron- and vitamin-deficient diet the women consumed. There are holes in this explanation and the last word on Plummer-Vinson syndrome and cancer of the pharynx and esophagus in Sweden isn't in yet, I'm sure. Needless to say, though, researchers have watched the falling rates of these cancers with great interest. Clearly, *certain dietary changes can turn old cancer patterns upside down.*

Most cancers in the United States are not related to vitamin deficiencies, mainly because we are not a malnourished population. The standard American diet may leave much to be desired, but the big problem for all but the very poorest among us is *excess.* The truth is, with a few exceptions (more about them below), anyone who gets fifteen hundred or more calories a day in a reasonable mix of fruits, vegetables, cereal grains and meat is practically guaranteed adequate amounts of all vital nutrients. And "adequate" is enough. Though our national tendency has always been to equate more with better, the person who gets two, three or more times the minimum daily requirement of vital nutrients isn't necessarily two or three times as healthy as the person who gets "just enough." A look at the big picture tells all: more vitamins are sold in the United States than in any other place in the world, yet we have no epidemiological evidence to suggest that they protect us from cancer or any of the other major killer diseases afflicting our population.

There are exceptions: pregnant women may need supplemental vitamins. People who are on strict dietary regimens for health reasons may also benefit from additional vitamins and minerals. (The man or woman on an ulcer diet, for example, may need supplemental amounts of vitamin C and the B-complex group.) Vitamins may help during periods of stress when a person is not eating well. Growing children and the elderly, whose diets may not meet their needs, usually need additional vitamins and minerals.

Heavy smokers tend to have low levels of vitamin C. No one knows whether this is universally true, or even whether it is significant. Nevertheless, smokers probably should make an extra effort to get additional vitamin C either in their food or in capsule or tablet form. (Also, as I mentioned earlier, because of the epithelial damage caused by smoking, they probably should also increase their vitamin A intake somewhat.) People who are moderate to heavy drinkers are often advised to get more of the B-complex vitamins.

Then there are those people who say they simply "feel better" when they take vitamins. I won't argue with the way they feel. In the long run, a few dollars a month is a small price to pay for "feeling better," and the fact is, most vitamins are apparently harmless even when taken in very large doses. (Vitamins A and D are the exceptions.) Any amounts of them that the body cannot use are excreted with the urine. (It's been said that the Hudson River has more vitamins in it than any body of water in the world.) But I can assure you that ten to fifteen miles a week in a walking or jogging or running program will do far more than all the vitamins in town to make you feel better—and will yield some real medical benefits as well.

I also question the faddish belief that enormous doses of vitamins—"megavitamins"—are a cure-all or preventive for all of our modern ailments. I'll even go one step further and say that anyone who tries to tell you that megavitamins will cure or prevent disease, especially cancer, is poorly informed.

I don't mean to imply that vitamins and minerals are unimportant. On the contrary, they're crucial to good health and cancer-protective eating. As we've seen, deficiencies are linked to certain kinds of cancer, so it's obvious that we must all make an effort to get *enough* of the vital nutrients. But once again, nutritional excess is a bigger problem for most Americans, and megavitamins are just one more excess. And one for which we probably do not know all of the complications.

18

A Few Words about
Organic Farming

I may as well make clear right here at the beginning where I stand on the subject of organic farming. Organically produced fruits and vegetables, when sold because of their "purity" at prices well over those charged for ordinary produce, are among the largest public rip-offs of the 1970s. Now don't misunderstand me. Health food stores serve a definite purpose—they offer a choice of specialty foods such as buckwheat flour and whole wheat spaghetti. Raw, salt-free cashews can be purchased there for the person on a low-salt diet, and where else can you buy the chocolate substitute carob? For the person on a special diet health food stores are indeed helpful. However, I would suggest you not rely on them for the medical advice which most make readily available (in many instances, it seems, they are more interested in selling their large volume of vitamins than in supplying special foods) or for organically grown produce.

The primary idea behind organic farming is to grow food "naturally" without the use of chemical fertilizers and insecticides, in as pure an environment as possible. It's a worthy aspiration, and the organic farmer who is committed to that ideal certainly would not be guilty of deliberately using commercial chemical products on his crops. But hard as it is to face the fact, there is no way that he can avoid *some* outside chemical contact with his produce through wind-blown dust and rainfall. Total isolation is impossible and actually not necessary, even if emotionally desirable. It has been suggested to the United States Congress that in the interest of honesty the terms "natural" and "organic" be prohibited from advertising.

In the section on food additives and contaminants, I mentioned that certain fertilizers and insecticides were banned by the federal government because they had been proven carcinogenic in tests with laboratory animals. (Some others are what we call "mutagenic," which means that they are capable of altering the chromosomes of animals to which they are administered.) By and large, the really dangerous compounds have been taken off the market already; many others remain under investigation. But remember: no human cancers are known to result from these compounds.

I have also explained that many insecticides still in use are "stable" compounds. This means that instead of decomposing and being broken down into their chemical components on exposure to air, sunlight and water over a period of time, they linger on in the environment as they are. They are also "recycled." The insecticide intended for wheat in Kansas may return to the earth in rainfall over Nebraska cornfields—or on the garden plot where the organic farmer tends his tomatoes.

As for the organic farmer's concern about man-made chemical fertilizers with nitrates, he should be aware that the nitrate level in vegetables depends more on the kind of vegetable he is growing than on the nitrate level of the soil in which it is grown. Some kinds of vegetables will absorb high levels of nitrate from the soil regardless of whether the farmer uses man-made chemical fertilizers or organic manure. (As a matter of fact, before the plant can use it at all, any fertilizer must be broken down to an inorganic form.)

Nitrates, in any event, are not dangerous to human beings. Nitrites are what we should be most concerned about. Harmless nitrates within a plant are changed to nitrites gradually, when produce is improperly stored and loses its freshness.

My father used to say that an ear of corn picked before 10:00 A.M. wasn't fit to eat by lunchtime. Of course, he was referring to corn's rapid loss of fresh-picked flavor and as far as I know, he had little awareness of things like nitrates and nitrites. I have friends with gardens who start the water boiling first, *then* run out to the back to pick the corn. Their primary concern is also flavor. One of the advantages of growing vegetables at home is being able to get that fresh-picked flavor every time. Gardening is also a good, relaxing hobby. And who knows, the day may come when, as our planet becomes more and more heavily populated, we will all have to return to raising some of our own food on any small plot of land that can be made available.

But the important thing is this: there is practically no way to tell the difference, nutritionally or otherwise, between a mature, fresh, good-quality organically grown tomato and a mature, fresh, good-quality commercially grown tomato. Since this is so, it makes little sense to pay a premium price for the "organic" tomato.

Since you can't tell by looking or tasting, and since there is no way to identify, control and inspect organic growers and processors, it is reasonable to suspect that at least some of the time "organic" vegetables are simply taken from the bushel basket headed for the supermarket and rerouted to the health food store, where they will be sold at a premium.

19

Why Nuts Are Overrated

What we call nuts are really single-celled fruits enclosed in a shell. Most grow on trees. Peanuts are an exception; there is usually more than one within the shell and they grow on small plants. They also derive some nitrogen from the air, so they're sometimes grouped, along with soybeans, peas and beans as legumes.

The different kinds of nuts vary so much in the calories they supply, as well as in their protein and fat content, that it seems more convenient to include a table rather than attempt a type-by-type discussion. In general—with the exception of chestnuts and water chestnuts—nuts are low in carbohydrates and high in calories, fat and protein. Peanuts are a particularly rich source of plant protein in which almost all of the essential amino acids are represented. (The 26 percent protein content indicated in Table 2 is for raw peanuts, however. Some of the protein and amino acids are lost in the roasting process.)

The really interesting thing about nuts is their very high ratio of polyunsaturated to saturated fatty acids—in walnuts and almonds it's twelve to one, with pecans a close runner up at eleven to one. Because of this ratio, which is very helpful in lowering cholesterol, physicians often recommend nuts as an occasional snack for people who are vulnerable to heart disease. (A few years ago it was quite the thing among doctors—especially heart specialists—to carry around with them small packages of walnuts to munch on.)

2. THE CONTENTS OF NUTS

	Calories per 100 gm.	% Protein per 100 gm.	% Fat per 100 gm.	Approximate Saturated to Polyunsaturated fats ratio
Almonds	598	19	54	1:12
Brazil nuts	654	14	67	1:5
Cashews	561	17	46	1:4
Filberts or hazelnuts	634	13	62	1:12
Peanuts	585	26	50	1:3
Pecans	687	9	71	1:11
Pistachios	594	19	54	1:7
Walnuts (black or English)	651	15	64	1:12

As you know by now, one of the primary aims of the Anti-Cancer Diet is to reduce consumption of fats of all kinds. Despite their cholesterol-lowering properties, nuts are so high in fat that I can't encourage you to eat them in quantity. If you have to choose between two high-fat foods, it's better to opt for the one with the more favorable ratio of polyunsaturated to saturated fats. But my general recommendation has to be to use nuts sparingly. An occasional sprinkle on a salad or cereal, a peanut butter (or other nut butter) sandwich once in a while, a handful of walnuts or almonds as a now-and-then snack are okay. Otherwise, avoid them.

A few final words about nuts: like cereal grains, improperly stored nuts make an ideal environment for the growth of the mold that produces the very potent carcinogen aflatoxin. Aflatoxin-contaminated nuts are thought to be a *direct* cause of liver cancer in some parts of Africa. As a result, consumer groups here have questioned the safety of nuts and nut products grown and processed in this country. Traces of the contaminant have been found in some of these products, but always in amounts that were considered too small to be of any danger to human health.

20

How Guilty Is Coffee?

We Americans stagger out of bed, fumble into our clothes and reach for a cup of coffee to kick us awake in the morning. Some of us feel that we can't get going without it. On mornings when we're too rushed for coffee we're inclined to say that the day is "off to a bad start."

Now good old coffee, our morning wake-up drink—and for many Americans the preferred beverage after every meal and for between-meal pick-me-ups as well—is not only becoming remarkably costly at this writing. It may well increase our cancer risk.

No, coffee is not a carcinogen. But it does look as though it plays a role as catalyst. In other words, like excessive amounts of alcohol, a heavy intake of coffee, in combination with other factors, appears to make the development of cancer more likely.

I'm a coffee drinker myself, and based on what I now know about the drink, I plan to keep my intake well under five cups a day. On most days I'll try to get by with only two cups. I'll avoid coffee *with* meals and have it either well before or well after my breakfast, lunch or dinner. I suggest you do the same.

One reason why you should consider modifying your coffee drinking habits has to do with the nitrite-amine reaction explained in chapter 16. If you remember, when substances containing nitrites and others containing amines are eaten together or are present in the stomach at the same time, they may combine to form nitrosamines. There's no doubt in anyone's mind that nitrosamines are carcinogens.

Not too long ago there were a few studies implying that nitrites and amines in the stomach would be so diluted by other food, water or whatever that the amount of nitrosamines formed by them would be insignificant. (Imagine combining a handful of baking soda and a cup of vinegar. Undiluted, the two would hiss and fizz into carbon dioxide and water. But mix them up in a full swimming pool and their reaction would be negligible.) Those studies were tremendously reassuring to those of us who had hoped that the nitrite-amine reaction would prove to be only a test tube concern with little significance in the lives of real people.

Then, in April of 1975, B. C. Challis and C. D. Bartlett, two organic chemists at the Imperial College in London, published a rather startling paper based on their attempts to discover any possibly carcinogenic effects of coffee consumption.

In short, the London chemists found that even when nitrites and amines were diluted in a large volume of liquid, the nitrosamine yield increased *tenfold* when as little as one-third of a cup of coffee was added to the solution.

Their findings call up unsettling visions of people all across the United States waking up, preceding their breakfasts with some kind of morning medication containing amines (a tranquilizer, perhaps, or an antihistamine or antibiotic); then sitting down to a meal that includes ham or bacon or some other high-nitrite food; then finally washing it all down with the catalyst—coffee. The result would be mass production in the stomach of carcinogenic nitrosamines.

The vision is unrelievedly gloomy save for one thing: orange juice or some other food high in vitamin C is a traditional accompaniment to breakfast in this country. And as I pointed out in the chapter on processed meats, vitamin C or ascorbic acid acts to prevent the nitrites and amines from combining into nitrosamines. (For this reason I've stressed the need to include a food rich in vitamin C with each and every meal.)

Now let's take a look at some of the other serious charges against coffee.

In reviewing the habits of bladder cancer patients living in the Boston area, Dr. Philip Cole of the Harvard School of Public Health, discovered an unusually large number of heavy coffee drinkers among them. The incidence of bladder cancer in coffee-drinking females appeared to be quite a bit higher than for non-coffee-drinking females. Men who drank coffee were at a moderately increased risk over men who did not.

Cole's 1971 study caused quite a furor. If a sound correlation could be established between coffee drinking and bladder cancer, then the public had to be warned.

There are problems in conducting any kind of study, but collecting and interpreting statistical data on human beings is the trickiest of all. For example, many of Dr. Cole's subjects were smokers as well as coffee drinkers. We already know that there is an increased incidence of bladder cancer among smokers. (At first thought, this might appear to be an unlikely association, since the primary effects of tobacco smoke are on the respiratory system. However, certain extremely soluble chemicals in the smoke are excreted with the urine and some of those soluble chemicals have proved to be powerfully carcinogenic when administered to animals. When this is understood, the relationship between bladder cancer and smoking begins to make sense.)

To make a long story short, we still cannot be sure whether the significant factor in Dr. Cole's study was the coffee drinking or the smoking. Up until now, we've had no really conclusive study of bladder cancer in which coffee drinking and smoking were separated.

Dr. Irwin Bross, at Roswell Park Memorial Institute in Buffalo, attempted to regulate the two factors. His study, done in 1973, implies that coffee drinking is of little significance in the development of bladder cancer in women and only slightly increased the risk of bladder cancer in men.

Those are the two most important studies yet made, and neither is conclusive. For all that, however, let's not forget that among the Seventh-day Adventists, who neither smoke cigarettes nor drink coffee, the incidence of bladder cancer is 75 percent less than for the rest of us.

Here and there in the medical literature we find scattered bits of incriminating evidence concerning coffee and its relationship to other kinds of cancer. Most of it only raises more questions to be answered.

In 1973 a brief report in the *British Cancer Journal* indicated a correlation between coffee drinking and cancer of the kidney. The author's technique was to gather statistics on kidney cancer death rates in various countries and compare the figures with per capita coffee consumption. In some countries the relationship between the two factors was striking. But there were also some glaring discrepancies. For example, per capita coffee consumption in the United States is five to six times greater than in Great Britain, yet the study shows that the mortality rate from cancer of the kidney is only just slightly higher here than in England.

We have to conclude that if coffee drinking is indeed a factor in the development of cancer of the kidney, it is not on the basis of what we call a "dose relationship," where the more coffee consumed, the greater the risk of kidney cancer. Dose relationships are always important in assessing epidemiological studies—unless, of course, the agent in question (coffee, in this case) acts as a catalyst, not as a cause.

We feel that coffee's role in the development of cancers of the bladder and possibly the stomach and kidney may be just that—catalytic—but we still can't say with certainty how, or why, it works that way.

There's no doubt at all that too much coffee has other negative effects on the human body. Ulcer patients and people with hypertension (high blood pressure) do better on coffee-free diets. Minor gastrointestinal problems—"irritable bowel," stomach roars and gurgles, mild diarrhea—often improve when coffee intake is reduced.

More important, a study published in 1974 suggests that more than five cups of coffee a day increases your coronary heart disease risk. (The study came in for some words of criticism on the same basis as Cole's study on coffee drinking and bladder cancer: some of the coffee drinkers surveyed were also cigarette smokers.)

To sum up, coffee is a little like the criminal who's always being indicted but each time manages to escape conviction. We have ample reason to feel uneasy about unlimited coffee drinking but we still can't pin anything definite on it. That's why I say, if you enjoy it, keep on drinking it. But try to stay within that five-cup-a-day maximum, and time your coffee drinking away from meals.

21

A Warning about Tea

Tea in moderation is fine. Anyone who likes a spot of it with toast at breakfast or as a midafternoon pick-me-up can safely carry on as before. I do want to urge you to drink tea at reasonable temperatures, however. If it scalds your throat on the way down, it's too hot to handle.

You may be surprised to learn that tannin, one of the components of tea that gives it its characteristic "tealike" flavor (and which is used in other forms to convert animal hides into leather), is known to be a very weak carcinogen. When administered in large doses, tannin induces tumors in experimental animals.

Why, then, do I say that it's safe to continue drinking tea in moderation? Because when we look at the incidence of cancer around the world, we find that no particular form of the disease correlates with heavy tea drinking. The English—the world's most prodigious tea drinkers—in their enthusiasm go through tea leaves at the rate of about nine pounds per person per year. Several Oriental populations love their tea almost as much. We in the United States are not so avid; we sip it at the rate of a pound of leaves per person per year. If the tannin in tea caused cancer in humans, we would certainly see a similar pattern of tumor incidence in England and parts of the Orient, with a smaller incidence of the same kind of tumor in the United States. We don't. The truth is, there is nothing in the large-scale geographical distribution of cancer that incriminates tea.

Now I'll do another one of those seeming about-faces and point out a few studies, done on smaller, local scales, which indicate that certain variations in the way tea is consumed are linked to certain kinds of cancer.

In Japan there are some fairly well-defined areas of the country with an exceptionally high rate of cancer of the esophagus. There are other nearby areas where the disease is much more rare. Epidemiologists are immediately interested when they catch wind of such local variations in the cancer rate. Sponsored by a National Cancer Institute grant, Dr. Mitsuo Segi of the Aichi Cancer Center in Japan studied the situation and in April, 1975, reported that the unusually high rate of cancer has to do with the local consumption of a mixture that can best be described as "tea gruel."

The tea gruel fancier makes it by packing tea leaves tightly into a cotton pouch and then boiling the pouch in water. After boiling, rice is added to the pouch and it is boiled again. When done, the rice is a drinkable tea-flavored mush that is customarily swallowed at temperatures near boiling.

Other regional associations between tea drinking and cancer of the esophagus crop up in the medical literature. For instance, there's a high incidence of the disease in some parts of India where tea gruel is unknown but where tea is taken at extremely high temperatures.

What are we to make of findings such as these? Well, it's believed that the tannins—mild carcinogens, let's not forget—are more reactive at high temperatures. (An alternate theory has it that contact with extreme heat damages the lining of the esophagus, making it more vulnerable to possibly carcinogenic influences such as the tannin in the tea.)

That's why I say that though tea drinking in moderation is perfectly harmless, it's a good idea to choose iced tea, or to allow hot tea to cool somewhat before swallowing it.

One more thing you should know about tea: a team of South African investigators and researchers from the University of Washington did some experimental work on gastrointestinal absorption. They found that a very high tea intake tended to affect the process by which the body absorbs iron from food, often creating a situation that could lead to iron-deficiency anemia. In the chapter on alcohol you'll see that iron deficiencies are linked with gastrointestinal cancers.

But as I've already pointed out, it's doubtful that iron deficiency alone, or alcohol alone, or anything alone (save for the most potent carcinogens) causes cancers. More and more, in trying to solve the puzzles cancer poses for us, we see the disease less as having a single, simple cause and more as the result of two, three or more imbalances.

22

What about Alcohol?

Is the Anti-Cancer Diet a drinking man's diet? Is it okay to order a cocktail at lunch and sip a glass or two of wine at dinner in the evening? What about chugging down a couple or more beers in front of the tv set each night?

I wish I could say outright either no, there is no relationship between alcohol and cancer, so you can let your drinking be limited only by how much you enjoy it and how much you can hold; or yes, there *is* a link, so scratch alcohol off your list completely. Unfortunately I can't. There is an alcohol-cancer connection, but it's neither direct nor clear. Though there's no good evidence indicating that drinking moderate amounts of alcohol causes cancer, there is reason to believe that drinking in combination with certain other factors results in conditions that set the stage for the development of the disease.

Therefore, I'm going to urge you to limit your drinking. If you're serious about wanting to increase your chances of living a long, cancer-free life, I'm going to suggest that you consume no more than sixty cc's—or about two ounces—of alcohol per day. That amounts to four mixed drinks or cocktails per day (assuming each drink is made with an ounce of 90 proof liquor) OR one half bottle of wine OR three cans of beer. We're concerned about actual alcohol content, and 90 proof whiskey is 45 percent alcohol.

To get a better idea of the alcohol-cancer connection, let's invent an imaginary character and call him Jack. Then let's consider some of the different ways that drinking could increase Jack's risk of developing cancer.

We don't need to know much about Jack. But for convenience' sake, let's say he's a man in his middle forties with a high-pressure sales job. Part of his drinking is done at business lunches and dinners at which he entertains clients. He's also likely to come home at night and have two or three more drinks to unwind from the tensions of the day. It's not unusual for Jack to consume seven ounces of alcohol in all over a twenty-four-hour period. (It doesn't matter what kinds of drinks Jack favors; what matters is the *amount* of alcohol itself.)

Jack is also a smoker. In this country, something like 90 percent of cancers of the mouth and larynx occur in smokers. Of course, all smokers do not develop the disease. But as a person who smokes *and* drinks, Jack is more than twice as likely to become a victim of one of these cancers as the nondrinker. The odds are similar for cancer of the esophagus. Some cancer experts go so far as to say that without alcohol, the incidence of cancer of the mouth, larynx and esophagus in the United States would fall by about 50 percent.

If Jack does develop one of those cancers, would we be right in saying that his drinking caused the disease? No, not exactly. But drinking probably made him a much easier target for the carcinogens in tobacco smoke.

They used to say, "If you drink, don't drive." To which we now have to add "or smoke." Better yet, cut way back on both.

There are other ways that excessive drinking could increase Jack's cancer risk. For example, after years of belting them down, Jack will be far more susceptible to pancreatitis than the average nondrinker. In the medical lexicon, any condition ending with the suffix *itis* indicates the presence of inflammation (as in appendicitis and bursitis). The pancreas is a gland that nestles within the first loop of the small intestine. It secretes insulin directly into the bloodstream and delivers fluids essential to the digestive process to the upper intestine. Apparently the pancreas of the person who drinks large amounts of alcohol becomes more easily inflamed. In examining the pancreases of heavy drinkers, pathologists have noted changes in the lining of the ducts. Some of these changes are the kind we call "premalignant"—which means that though cancer is not yet present it may not be far off. Add to that the 1968 findings of Drs. G. E. Burch and A. Ansari in New Orleans that 65 percent of their patients with carcinomas of the pancreas had been moderate to heavy drinkers, and it begins to look as though Jack has another good reason to cut back on his alcohol consumption.

Again, if Jack got cancer of the pancreas, it wouldn't be precisely accurate to say it was because he drank too much. But alcohol might have affected his pancreas in such a way that it became more vulnerable to environmental carcinogens when they came along.

What if Jack's drinking becomes a *real* problem? What if he joins the ranks of those ten million other Americans who can properly be called "alcoholics"? What if his problem gets so out of hand that he becomes one of the 10 to 15 percent of alcoholics who develop cirrhosis of the liver? (The percentage of cirrhotic alcoholics is greater for some reason in other countries than here.)

It's a medical axiom that the cirrhotic who lives long enough eventually succumbs to hepatoma, a relatively rare and virtually incurable form of liver cancer. Most cirrhotics don't live that long. In this country hepatoma claims fewer than five thousand lives each year.

But suppose Jack does die of hepatoma. Was it because of his drinking? Strictly speaking, no. But it's highly unlikely that he would have been a victim of liver cancer if he hadn't been cirrhotic. And if he hadn't been a heavy drinker he probably wouldn't have developed cirrhosis.

Alcohol, like all the other foods and beverages we've considered so far, is not carcinogenic. But we have good reason to suspect that it's involved in the cancer process in ways other than the ones just mentioned.

Our friend Jack, for example, might drink heavily and never become an alcoholic, but his high alcohol intake could result in any of a number of vitamin and mineral deficiencies. We are not quite sure how this happens, but we know that alcohol tends to interfere with the liver's function as storage vat and dispenser of essential nutrients. An out-of-kilter liver might result in a thiamine deficiency, which in turn could lead to disorders of the central nervous system. Or there could be deficiencies of magnesium and zinc that could cause cardiovascular and kidney problems. But most important insofar as cancer is concerned is that heavy drinking can result in chronic iron deficiency, one consequence of which can be premalignant lesions—tissue abnormalities—of the gastrointestinal tract.

Jack's overdrinking could wreak havoc with his body's immune system, making him generally more vulnerable to the disease. As I've pointed out earlier, cancer experts are in agreement that there are varying levels of susceptibility to the disease, that some people are simply more cancer-resistant than others in much the same way that some people have more allergies or "catch cold" more easily than others. A high alcohol intake over a period of years does seem to alter the drinker's immunity, but how important the change is and whether it does indeed make a person less cancer-resistant is not known. Some researchers believe that the most important link in the alcohol-cancer connection has to do with the effects of alcohol on the immune system.

What does it all add up to? Enough to urge Jack or anyone who is a really heavy drinker to cut back or stop. (That, I know, may be an impossible undertaking for true alcoholics, and the best advice anyone can give to them is to suggest they seek social and medical advice.) As for the moderate drinker, he or she should take care not to exceed the limits indicated at the beginning of this chapter. For good health, alcohol has little to recommend it.

23

What to Do about Soft Drinks

Soft drinks come in two categories: the kind made with sugar and the other kind, sometimes called diet soda, made with sugar substitutes.

Aside from water, the major ingredient in regular soft drinks is sugar. No scientific study has ever indicated that sugar is carcinogenic or that there is a direct link between sugar and cancer. But sugar contributes only calories to human nutrition. I suppose that people who don't get enough calories benefit by drinking soft drinks. But they'd benefit even more by eating greater amounts of more nutritious food. Very few Americans have a deficiency of calories.

In sugar-free soft drinks saccharin has been the major flavoring ingredient. (The cyclamates, another group of noncaloric sweeteners that were in common use several years ago, were banned, not so much because they were thought to be carcinogenic, but because it was feared they might be "mutagenic," and cause damage to the genes.)

It has been proposed that saccharin be banned as of this writing, and there is every reason to believe it will be. In chapter 1 I explained my disapproval of this ban, but realize it was necessary under our current laws. These laws need revision and only public pressure will bring it about. I know of no evidence that saccharin has produced tumors of any kind in humans. Of course it seems reasonable to suggest that saccharin not make up 5 percent (by weight) or even .5 percent of your diet. However, these arguments are academic unless public pressure can cause the FDA to rescind its ban on saccharin. And there is also always the hope that some other sugar substitute can be made available.

Coloring agents—dyes—are present in both kinds of soft drinks. Most of them are on the GRAS list. There is some doubt about the safety of others, particularly the notorious Red #2. At government request, this dye is being phased out of use. It added nothing but color, and if it can be replaced by a less questionable substance—or even if it can't and the soft drinks and other food to which it was added lose eye appeal—its withdrawal from use will make many people feel more at ease about the safety of their food. It would seem that the withdrawal of Red Dye #2 is based on evidence generally similar to that which resulted in the withdrawal of saccharin. However, the difference here is that a coloring agent serves only a cosmetic purpose. Its loss should hurt no one. Taking saccharin from the diabetic and from those who are trying to control their weight results in an unfortunate hardship.

My soft drink recommendations should be obvious: consumption of regular soft drinks containing sugar should be regulated by your need for calories or your ability to tolerate calories. If too many calories are your problem and sugar-free soft drinks are available, then only use in excess can be construed as dangerous.

24

The Sugar Story

Sugar has come under a lot of fire lately. Recent books condemn it as the source of many of our modern-day ills. It's undoubtedly true that most Americans eat more highly refined sugar products than is good for them. In fact, we probably don't need to eat any foods that have sugar as an added ingredient because almost everything we consume, from the most complex proteins and fats to the simpler carbohydrates, is converted to a sugar—dextrose—before our bodies can make use of it for energy. It also seems logical that if sugar per se were truly harmful, the human body would have evolved in ways that enabled it to make use of some other substance as its "universal fuel."

The one connection between sugar and cancer is a tenuous one and is the result of very high levels of the substance in the blood. When blood sugar is elevated and stays relatively high, sugar may be spilled into the urine, and diabetes is the result. Diabetes always carries with it other disease risks. The diabetic, for example, is at greater risk for arteriosclerosis, coronary artery disease and, as we've seen, certain kinds of cancer—most notably cancer of the uterus.

I'm going to suggest that you cut back on your consumption of candy, pastries and other sugary treats—not because sugar is a particularly sinister foodstuff, but because eating less of it will help you keep your blood sugar level within the normal range. It will also help you keep your weight down where it belongs.

At four calories per gram, sugar supplies a lot of calories but practically nothing else. It's pure carbohydrate, with no fat, no protein and no fiber. Some authors and food faddists make a distinction between various kinds of sugar, implying that there is something peculiarly unhealthful about the kind you buy in a box at the supermarket. Honey, they say, is preferable.

Honey may indeed be better suited to specific uses (give me honey on toast instead of sugar any day) but for health the two are practically identical. Refined white cane sugar is a simple sugar called sucrose. Honey is another very simple sugar called fructose. They have the same number of calories per gram, and in fact the major difference between the two is that the first is processed by mechanical means and the second is processed by bees.

Some recent research indicates that fructose might play an even bigger part in raising triglyceride levels in the blood than sucrose. This is important information. Elevated serum triglycerides may be a factor in the development of coronary artery disease—a factor that in some people could be as significant as elevated serum cholesterol levels. Therefore, some of the criticism aimed at refined white sugar applies at least equally to honey. Very probably, consumed in moderation, neither of these foods is quite as bad as it's made out to be.

25

How to Cook the Anti-Cancer Way

I've no wish to write a cookbook. But while some food is totally unobjectionable from an Anti-Cancer point of view, the manner in which it is prepared adds a definite element of danger. Therefore, I think we have to go into safe methods of preparation or cooking versus the kind that can increase the risk of malignant disease.

In this regard Japan offers still another striking illustration. In Japan, remember, there is a much higher rate of stomach cancer than we have here. Studies give us reason to believe that among the Japanese, men and women who eat large quantities of pickled vegetables and dried salt fish run a greater stomach cancer risk than others in the population. At the same time we know that simply eating great amounts of *un*processed vegetables and fish has either no correlation or a negative correlation with the development of the disease. This has led researchers to suspect that there is something about the manner of preparation of these two food items—pickled vegetables and dried salt fish—that makes eating them an additional cancer risk factor.

As it turns out, the crude salt commonly used in Japan in pickling brine and to process salt fish contains relatively high levels of nitrites. It is generally believed that Japanese salt, with its high sodium nitrite content, is at least partially responsible for the high rate of stomach cancer among the Japanese. (It's worth noting that of the Japanese men and women studied, the ones who ate greater than usual amounts of certain vegetables such as celery, corn and lettuce, as well as cauliflower and broccoli, which are cruciferous vegetables, had a reduced stomach cancer risk. This may be because these people are getting in their diets more of the vitamin C that blocks the nitrite-amine reaction that could lead to stomach cancer. Or it could be that these vegetables, especially the cruciferous ones, are indeed cancer-protective to human beings.)

Studies done in Iceland, Norway and the United States yield similar findings. Again, there seems to be an increased risk of stomach cancer among those who eat large amounts of smoked and salted fish, and a reduced risk when consumption of certain vegetables is high. The salt used in the United States is not high in nitrates, but nitrates and nitrites *are* used in processed fish and meat to prevent the growth of the organisms that cause botulism. This may explain the higher incidence of stomach cancer among those who consume large quantities of these products.

In any event, the point is not that salt promotes cancer in the United States (though most of us probably use too much of it and would benefit by learning to relish food that is unsalted or only very lightly salted), nor that fish is a bad food (it's an excellent food). The point is: what we do with our food before we eat it may be as important as the food itself.

Smoked meats certainly warrant some consideration when the data from Japan so strongly incriminate the combination of smoking and excessive salting of food. Chemical analysis of the surfaces of smoked meats indicate the presence of compounds called "polynuclear hydrocarbons." Some of these are carcinogenic to animals. However, simply by covering the meat with a few layers of cloth while it is being smoked, meat processors can virtually eliminate the suspect hydrocarbons. Meat prepared this way is safe—at least as far as polynuclear hydrocarbons are concerned—and still has the traditional savory smoked flavor.

Real smoking is usually done commercially rather than in the home. Smoke flavorings, the liquid kinds that come in bottles and can be added to various foods cooked in the home, are apparently harmless. The distillate "smokes" now on the market have passed a number of chemical and biological tests, and these products are on the government's GRAS list.

Charcoal broiling, a method of cooking that has become an enjoyable backyard pastime for millions of suburbanites, is another matter. Whenever cancer and cooking are discussed together, the question of whether charcoal broiling is safe or not comes up.

Research in this area is several years old, and the subject needs to be investigated further. However, in one of the studies I was able to locate, a group of scientists took fifteen steaks, each weighing about one kilo (or 2.2 pounds), and charbroiled them to the equivalent of well-done. An analysis of the surface areas of the meat did indeed indicate the presence of some dangerous compounds, among them benzo(a)pyrene.

Benzo(a)pyrene is believed to be one of the cancer-causing components of cigarette smoke. The eight micrograms of benzo-(a)pyrene found in a kilo of steak is the equivalent of the benzo-(a)pyrene in the smoke of approximately *six hundred* cigarettes.

In charcoal broiling, food is exposed to smoke and subjected to very high surface temperatures. The most likely source of benzo-(a)pyrene is the liquefied fat from the meat, which drips down onto the hot coals and is "pyrolized" (chemically changed by heat). The smoke resulting from this reaction rises and permeates the meat above it.

Until more becomes known about this method of cooking and the chemical carcinogens that result, my recommendation on charcoal broiling is: *limit it.* Oven broiling or roasting, in which the fat does not drip down onto hot coals and benzo(a)pyrene is not produced, seem much safer (though admittedly less idyllic) means of preparing meat than on an outdoor barbecue grill.

If you're very reluctant to discontinue backyard or patio charcoal broiling, then by all means take the precaution of trimming all visible fat from the meat before placing it on the grill. Anyone who's tried charcoal broiling a steak or burger knows that at times there is practically no smoke and at other times fatty drippings cause billows of smoke to rise. When you see smoke beginning to rise, remove the meat from the grill and wait until the smoking stops before you replace it. It may take longer to charbroil meat in this way, but the benzo(a)pyrene content of the finished steak will be less than if you'd cooked it without taking this precaution.

As for the safety of charbroiling fowl, frankfurters and other meats, there are no studies available so far. But the problem would certainly seem to be much the same as in charbroiling steaks and hamburgers. One way to get around the problem in chicken and turkey would be to remove the skin—where concentrations of benzo(a)pyrene would be greatest—before eating. (Since most of the fat in poultry is in or just under the skin, it's a good idea to remove it regardless of how the bird has been cooked.)

Fats—the kind used in cooking, not the kind found in meat and poultry—also need to be considered. To begin with, frying is the least desirable of all cooking techniques since it invariably adds more fat to the food. This is bad enough even when the cooking fat is an unsaturated one such as corn oil. But when a saturated fat such as lard is used, cholesterol enters the picture as well. In general, then, don't fry if you can broil, bake, roast, steam or boil.

If for some reason you feel you must continue to fry foods, make sure you don't use the same fat over and over again. Reusing cooking fats and oils is a common practice in many households, restaurants and industrial food processing plants. Even when an unsaturated fat is used to start with, repeated use tends to shift its chemical composition more and more toward saturation. Most studies indicate that an unsaturated fat must be heated to high temperatures—above 424° Fahrenheit, or 200° Celsius—at least eight or ten times before any significant shift toward saturation occurs, so in this sense reusing an oil only two or three times is "safe." Once again, though, it's safer still to choose some other cooking method and to avoid fried foods in restaurants, where you have no control over the kind of fat used or the number of times it's been reused.

Another point to keep in mind has to do with temperature. In general, the lower the temperature to which fats are heated, the less chance that polynuclear hydrocarbons will be formed. Slow cooking over low heat is preferable to shorter periods of cooking over intense heat.

Up to now we've been concerned primarily with cooking processes that can add new and dangerous substances to food. We also have to be concerned about cooking in ways that do not destroy cancer-protective vitamins and other desirable nutrients. Because overcooking can lower the nutritional value of some foods, a few extremists recommend that most things be eaten raw. We cook food to make it easier to eat and because some foods taste better cooked than raw. Cooking also kills bacteria. (Refrigeration prevents the rapid growth of these organisms, but only adequate cooking renders them harmless.) In addition, some foods need to be cooked in order to destroy chemically blocking elements (the soybean, discussed in chapter 15, is a good example). So despite the advice of some food faddists, most of us will continue to cook most of what we eat, and for good reason.

How to cook without overcooking and destroying vitamins is the real issue here. Good cooking methods depend on which vitamins we're trying to preserve. Vitamins are generally divided into two groups: fat-soluble (the ones that will dissolve in fat) and water-soluble (the ones that will dissolve in water). The fat-soluble vitamins are A, D, E and K. The least important of these in terms of what we now know about cancer prevention are D, E and K. These are all fairly stable and are neither destroyed nor lost when food is cooked in ordinary ways at the usual temperatures. Vitamin K is destroyed by contact with acids or alkali. Vitamins D and E are harmed by heavy exposure to ultraviolet rays.

Vitamin A is the least stable of the fat-soluble vitamins and also the most important one in cancer prevention. Exposure to air, excessive dryness and/or heat all have a detrimental effect on this vitamin. Though most cooking temperatures do not totally destroy vitamin A in food (vitamin A content is roughly comparable in carrots that are raw or cooked and the same is true of sweet potatoes), it's good to keep in mind that the higher the temperature, the more rapidly this vitamin deteriorates. Maximum amounts of vitamin A can be retained when food is cooked and eaten soon after it's purchased and stored in the meantime under refrigeration.

The water-soluble vitamins are vitamin C and the entire B-complex group. Of all vitamins, C—also called ascorbic acid—deteriorates most rapidly on exposure to heat and air. Alkaline substances are distinctly harmful to this vitamin, which means that it is destroyed if baking soda or other compounds containing an alkali are added during cooking. Vitamin C is extremely soluble in water and dissolves out of some vegetables during the first few minutes of cooking, though produce with a high acid content—tomatoes, for example—lose much less vitamin C on being cooked than nonacid foods such as potatoes.

Here are a few pointers for retaining the vitamin C content of various foods during cooking. First, use the least possible amount of water and cook for the shortest possible time. (Happily, most vegetables taste best when they're served still slightly crisp.) Don't shell peas, cut beans or peel any vegetable until just before cooking. In general, chop or cut vegetables as little as possible. Keep in mind that baked, boiled or steamed potatoes retain far more vitamin C if cooked whole. Fresh fruits lose vitamin C far more rapidly when stored at room temperature, and this is even more true of vegetables, so keep all fresh produce in the refrigerator. Quick freezing has little or no effect on vitamin C content, but the vitamin is quickly lost upon thawing. Therefore, frozen fruits should be served immediately after thawing, while frozen vegetables should be plunged directly into simmering water (or other cooking liquid) upon removal from the freezer.

In general, the same cooking and storing techniques that preserve the vitamin C content of food also prevent the loss of the B-complex vitamins. There are a few exceptions, however.

Thiamine, also called vitamin B_1, is only slightly more stable than vitamin C and, like C, is destroyed by alkaline substances added during cooking. The longer the cooking time and the more water used, the greater the loss of thiamine. Sometimes as much as 35 percent of this vitamin gets dumped out with the cooking water. Thiamine in cereal grains is more easily retained mainly because grains are usually baked or otherwise cooked slowly and at moderate temperatures. About 15 percent of the thiamine in wheat flour and other cereal grains is lost during baking, while more thiamine is lost from meat because most meats are cooked at higher temperatures.

Riboflavin (vitamin B_2) is not usually destroyed at standard cooking temperatures, nor is it very much affected by acids or exposure to air. It does deteriorate rapidly on exposure to light. Milk, an important source of riboflavin, should therefore either be stored in cartons or in dark glass bottles. (This is one reason why the clear milk bottle has all but disappeared.)

Some of the other B-complex vitamins—niacin, vitamin B_6 and vitamin B_{12} to be exact—are also relatively impervious to the usual range of cooking temperatures. Pantothenic acid, folic acid and biotin are not; they are also affected by alkaline substances added to the food. However, since they're found so abundantly in so many different foodstuffs that a deficiency of any of them is unlikely, and since there is little or no connection that we know of between them and the development of cancer, I won't elaborate further on techniques for preserving them. Suffice it to say that the same methods that prevent the deterioration and loss of vitamin C also tend to maintain the B-complex vitamins in food.

Within the last three or four years two new cooking techniques have become popular. One is the use of a slow cooker, sometimes called a "crock pot," and the other is the microwave oven. Surprisingly little is known about how these methods of cooking affect the nutritional value of food and, by extension, our health.

With the slow cooker, food is cooked at relatively low temperatures and very little if any cooking liquid is lost. This sounds ideal, but—and it's a very big but—since the cooking time is extended over a number of hours, much of the vitamin A and C in slow-cooked food can be destroyed. Unfortunately, as of now there are no studies to confirm or disprove this vitamin loss.

As for microwave ovens, material published by the manufacturers of these appliances suggest that they're the best thing that ever happened to food. However, when I asked for more specific nutritional data, one company representative told me there was none, the past studies were outdated because the firm was now producing a new improved model that operated on a wavelength different from the old.

Information from an appliance manufacturer always tends to be somewhat prejudiced in favor of the appliance, of course, but other information on microwave ovens, although available, is hard to find. However, material from the Home Economics Department at the University of Missouri and from Colorado State University is encouraging. It indicates that with microwave cooking the vitamin C in vegetables is retained better than with conventional cooking methods. This is partly because no water is used. There is also better retention of thiamine and riboflavin in beef. The tentative conclusion is that microwave cooking is at least equal to, and possibly better than, conventional cooking for preserving the vitamin content of food.

None of the studies I've reviewed have demonstrated that polynuclear hydrocarbons are formed in meats cooked by microwave. Since the actual temperatures used are relatively low, it's logical to assume that these compounds are not formed. Some tests indicate that the ratio of unsaturated to saturated fats does not change as a result of microwave cooking. Total fat content generally drops with cooking by any method, but fat loss was less with microwave cooking than conventional methods. Cholesterol levels in beef patties were also higher when cooked with microwave techniques, but not much.

At this point it appears that the microwave oven provides a convenient way of preparing food and is no more damaging to nutritional values than the old ways.

What about the damage microwaves might do to *us?* Some criticism has been directed at these appliances because we tend to equate microwaves with the more mysterious X rays and gamma rays. None of these wave energy forms leave a residue in food. We have found no dangerous residual products in food processed by them. All studies have shown the cooking effect on food to be due to heat generated, not to direct effect of microwave. As with X or gamma rays, microwaves should not be used on people except under very controlled conditions. Any harm from microwave ovens would seem to be related to accidental or careless operator exposure to the energy form rather than changes in the food.

PART
II

HOW TO FOLLOW
THE ANTI-CANCER
DIET

26

The Anti-Cancer Diet at a Glance

VEGETABLES—As much as you like. Choose as often as possible (preferably twice daily) from the cruciferous vegetables—cabbage, cauliflower, broccoli, spinach and turnips, among others —as well as celery and dill. These are the vegetables that reduce the incidence of tumor formation in laboratory animals and may have a similar effect in human beings. Vegetables provide the greatest amount of bulk when eaten raw and unpeeled.

FRUITS—Again, as much as you like. Fresh uncooked fruits are preferable. Apples, pears, peaches, apricots, plums and the like should be eaten with the peel.

CEREAL GRAINS—In general, eat more of the unrefined whole grain products. These include whole grain breakfast cereals such as oatmeal, all bran and shredded wheat, as well as whole wheat bread, brown rice, and bran to sprinkle on top of or mix in with pancake batter, muffins, meat loaf, soup, et cetera.

LEGUMES—Peas, beans (including soybeans) and peanuts can be used often. Their calorie content is moderate, their vitamin and mineral content is good, and they're excellent sources of vegetable protein. Dishes in which a legume is combined with a cereal grain provide high-quality complete protein and are a nice change of pace from animal protein.

RED MEAT—No more than six four-ounce servings per week of lean beef, pork, lamb or veal.

POULTRY—One or more four-ounce servings per week of chicken or turkey, skin removed. Ideally, chicken or turkey would be used to replace red meat for several meals during the week.

FISH—Two or more four-ounce servings of nonoily white-fleshed fish per week. Ideally, fish should be used to replace red meat at several meals.

PROCESSED MEATS—Ham, bacon, frankfurters, corned beef and many lunch meats not only have a high fat content but also contain nitrates and nitrites. Therefore, they have *no place* in the Anti-Cancer Diet. On those infrequent occasions when eating them is unavoidable, make sure to include a food high in vitamin C with the meal.

ORGAN MEATS—Liver, sweetbreads, kidneys, and brains are good sources of many vitamins and minerals but of all foods they're highest in cholesterol. Avoid them completely.

MILK—For adults, no more than two cups of *skimmed* milk per day.

CHEESE—To be used with discretion as a meat substitute. Skim milk cheeses are always preferable to whole milk varieties.

FATS AND OILS—Use as little as possible. When a fat or oil is necessary in cooking, choose corn oil margarine or liquid vegetable oil.

NUTS—High in vegetable protein and a good source of many vitamins and minerals, but unfortunately also too high in fat to be used in large amounts.

COFFEE—No more than five cups per day; coffee should be drunk before or between meals rather than as an accompaniment to the food.

TEA—No restriction, but never to be drunk scalding hot.

ALCOHOLIC BEVERAGES—No more than four one-ounce cocktails or mixed drinks per day (at an ounce of liquor per drink), or half a bottle of wine, or three cans of beer.

SOFT DRINKS—One or two bottles of dietetic (sugar-free) soda per day is fine. Regular soda (with sugar) should be avoided by people who must watch their weight, are diabetic or have elevated triglyceride levels.

CAKES, COOKIES, PASTRIES AND OTHER FOOD MADE WITH HIGHLY REFINED FLOUR AND SUGAR—To be avoided for several reasons. Their calorie content is high while they offer little in the way of nutritional value. (They're deficient in most vitamins and minerals, protein, fiber.) They also often contain large amounts of fat or oil. Angelfood cake is the exception. Choose fresh fruit, dried fruit, sherbet or gelatin desserts.

27

Get Your Fill of Cancer-Protective Vegetables—and Love It

As you now know, vegetables play a starring role in the Anti-Cancer Diet, with the cruciferous vegetables getting top billing. Assuming you're not going to drown them in butter or fry them or otherwise add unnecessary fat, eat as many cruciferous vegetables as you like; they're low in calories, bursting with vitamins and, best yet, their cancer-protective properties have already been demonstrated in laboratory animals.

Once again, here's a listing of the cruciferous vegetables in order of their effectiveness in inhibiting tumor growth in test animals:

Brussels sprouts
cabbage
broccoli
cauliflower
spinach
turnips
lettuce
celery
dill

With the exception of Brussels sprouts and turnips, all these vegetables are particularly delicious eaten chilled and raw, either in a salad or as part of a main course. Raw vegetables served with a dip made out of blender "sour cream" (recipe, page 234) or skim milk yogurt with herbs are an excellent appetizer as well.

The best way to cook vegetables is to steam them. Most of the vegetable dishes given in the meal-planning section of this book call for steaming. Steaming may take longer than boiling but for taste and texture the results are infinitely worth it, as you'll discover if you've never steamed a vegetable before.

To steam a vegetable, you need a double boiler or pot with tight-fitting cover. If you use a double boiler, water goes in the bottom part and the vegetables go in the top. Cover, allow the water to come to a boil, then cook until the vegetables reach the desired degree of tenderness. To steam vegetables in a large pot, you need a colander or rack or something to place the vegetables in so that they're suspended above the boiling water, not sitting right in it. When the water comes to a boil, cover and cook until the vegetables are tender. (If you're in the habit of eating very soft vegetables, try them a little crisper than usual. Remember: the less cooking time, the less vitamin loss.)

Some very good cooks add baking soda to vegetables as they cook in order to retain good color. This is unfortunate since baking soda destroys many vitamins.

To serve, squeeze a little lemon or lime juice over the vegetables, add parsley, chives or other herbs (paprika adds a nice color) and salt and pepper.

Remember, you can eat unlimited amounts of vegetables on the Anti-Cancer Diet—the more the better.

28

*How to Get More Fiber
into Your Diet*

Bran and a few other high-fiber foods are the superfoods of the moment. As we've seen, though fiber doesn't perform all the miracles that its most enthusiastic boosters claim for it, there are some very real benefits to be gained from eating more of the foods that add bulk to the diet. Many fruits and vegetables, eaten raw, peels and all, do just that. The same can be said for unrefined cereal grains, of which bran is only one.

The point is, bran isn't the *only* way to add fiber to a diet. It isn't even necessarily the best way. The following list will give you an indication of some of the wide range of *very* high-fiber foods that are readily available in the United States. All are at least 2 percent fiber. (Most fruits and vegetables, though they're excellent fiber sources, contain somewhat less. Highly refined and processed foods—commercial pastries, for example, and instant mashed potatoes—and most foods of animal origin contain little or no fiber.)

If you have some of the following foods occasionally and plenty of fresh fruits and vegetables every day, as recommended in the Anti-Cancer meal-planning section, your needs for fiber will be met in an entirely satisfactory way.

FOOD	PERCENT FIBER
dried almonds	2.6
dried uncooked apricots	3
raw blackberries	4.2
bran breakfast cereal	2
40% bran flakes	3.6
raisin bran	3
Brazil nuts	3.1
chick peas (garbanzos)	5.3
fresh or shredded coconut	4
fresh or dried dates	2.4
filberts (hazelnuts)	3
dried figs	5.6
raw guava	5.5
raw loganberries	3
cooked parsnips	2
dried uncooked peaches	3.1
roasted peanuts	2.4
fresh or frozen peas	2
pecans	2.3
raw black raspberries	5.1
raw red raspberries	3
soybean flour or grits	2.2
walnuts	2.1
whole wheat flour	2.3
wheat germ	2.5
puffed wheat	2

The beauty of bran (and probably one of the main reasons why Dr. David Reuben and others favor bran over all other high-fiber foods) is the fact that it can be combined easily with the other ingredients in almost any kind of recipe. That's because bran's rather bland flavor and innocuous texture don't interfere with the other flavors and textures in a dish. All it adds is bulk—and, of course, a few extra calories.

The pork and zucchini casserole (page 258) provides a good example of how bran can be added to a multiingredient main dish.

You might want to try adding bran (one fourth to one half cup) to some of your family's own casserole favorites. Of course, bran is a natural in muffins and bread. Two recipes that my wife, Ruth, and I particularly enjoy are the dilled brown muffins (page 242) and the oatmeal-applesauce bread (page 253). If you're an even moderately adventurous cook, why not add bran to some of the breads and muffins in your repertoire?

29

How to Dress a Salad

Most salad dressings have a base of oil or mayonnaise (which is mainly eggs and oil). Both kinds are undesirable on the Anti-Cancer diet. But salad greens—lettuce, spinach, escarole, endive, et cetera—are *highly* desirable. So what are your options?

First, you can make a very tasty fat-free salad by combining all the vegetables, squeezing a wedge or two of lemon or lime over them and tossing. Add salt and pepper (use a mill; freshly ground pepper tastes far better than the kind you sprinkle on from a shaker). Then a sprinkle of fresh or dried herbs. Choose from oregano, basil, dill, chives, and parsley to start with. Dried herbs should be crushed or crumpled in your hand before adding to release their full flavor and aroma. Don't forget either fresh garlic or garlic salt.

Skim milk yogurt can also be used as the base for a salad dressing. Simply add salt and pepper and herbs of your choice.

The blender "sour cream" recipe (page 234) is another mixture that can be used as the foundation of a salad dressing. Again, add herbs and seasonings of your choice.

Some commercially prepared salad dressings are unobjectionable. But before you buy, read labels and compare. Choose the kinds that contain no oil, no eggs, no cream or sour cream and no high-fat cheese.

In a restaurant, or as a dinner guest in a home where only a high-fat dressing is being served, you have little choice. Either eat the salad au naturel, or use the high-fat dressing *sparingly* so that it just barely moistens the vegetables.

30

How to Choose Lower-Risk Fats and Oils

The less fat of any kind you consume, the better off you're going to be. However, when you have to use small quantities of fats or oils for cooking, it's best to choose unsaturated vegetable products to avoid cholesterol.

The ingredients below are listed in descending order of preference: lowest-risk choices at the top, higher-risk choices at the bottom. In general, try to stay as close as possible to the top of the list.

BEST: Little or no fat or oil
Liquid vegetable oil, such as corn oil
Margarine, especially the kind mentioning liquid vegetable oil as its most prominent ingredient
Solid vegetable shortening

WORST: Butter and lard

Substitute vegetable oils for solid (hydrogenated) vegetable shortenings and butter when oiling pans for baking (better still, use nonstick pans) and for pan-broiling, frying, sautéing and browning food.

If you enjoy baking your own bread and pastries, seek out those cookbooks that provide recipes in which liquid vegetable oil is used in place of solid shortenings.

Whenever possible use corn oil margarine instead of butter. Better still, use neither.

Remember that all margarines are not alike. Some are made with large amounts of hydrogenated (solid) vegetable oil. These are not as desirable as the ones made primarily with liquid vegetable oil. Read labels, keeping in mind that the ingredients are listed in order of percentage used in the product. In other words, the first ingredient listed is present in greatest amount. Specifically, look for a margarine that has "liquid vegetable oil" (corn, safflower, peanut, soya, et cetera) as the first ingredient, with "partially hydrogenated" or "hardened polyunsaturated oil" as a secondary ingredient.

Whatever type of fat or oil you use, make it a habit to reduce the amount whenever possible. A tablespoon or so less fat or oil in a recipe often has no noticeable effect on the taste or texture of the final product.

31

How to Cut Back on Fat
by Using Nonstick Cookware

Nonstick cookware (Teflon is the brand name that comes first to most people's minds) is a real boon to the cook who wants to serve cancer-protective meals since muffin tins, cake and pie pans, cookie sheets, griddles, skillets and saucepans with a nonstick coating rarely need to be greased. If you're using this type of cookware, be aware that the oil or fat in a recipe may be included merely to prevent the food from sticking to the pot or pan. Ask yourself whether the fat can be reduced or eliminated. Often it can.

To date we have had no bad reports on Teflon or similar products.

32

Low-Risk Ways with Meat

Where there is meat there is always some fat and cholesterol. Since meat is a high-risk food, there may be somewhat less of it on the Anti-Cancer food plan than what you're used to. On the other hand, you might find that the amount of meat suggested in the menu plans that follow is not so very far from what you've been having all along, but that the methods of cooking and preparation are slightly different. Either way, if you've been eating the standard American diet, Anti-Cancer eating will probably be a bit of a novelty. But let me assure you that you needn't feel the least deprived. In fact, with the absence of heavy fats and thick gravies, the hearty taste and texture of the meat will come through better than ever before.

To get meat with more flavor and less fat, you have to begin at the beginning, at the store where you buy it. Rule number one is always to look for the cuts of meat with the least amount of fat. This may be difficult because many supermarkets package meats in ways that allow you to see only the front surface; too often what looks like lean sirloin from the front is extremely fatty from the back. Therefore, it may be a good idea to buy meat from a butcher. That way you can specify lean cuts and inspect your purchases before you leave the store. (I know that butcher shops have all but disappeared from certain areas of the country, but if there is one near you, it might be worthwhile to try buying there.)

If you're going to eat hamburger at all, it pays to buy a pound or so of good, lean round steak and have it ground for you rather than to invest in the "budget" hamburger that may be as much as 40 percent fat (which makes it less than a bargain after all).

Get into the habit of carefully trimming away *all* visible fat before cooking any cut of meat, and trim it again if necessary before eating.

As I mentioned earlier, the more well done the meat, the more fat will be cooked off and the less fat it will have when you eat it. This is true of virtually all meats. If you've always preferred rare steak and find the well-done kind not to your liking, then at least try a compromise and cultivate a taste for steaks cooked to *medium* doneness.

As we've seen, frying is probably the least desirable way of cooking just about anything—meat included—because it involves the use of additional fat.

Charcoal broiling is to be discouraged because of the polynuclear hydrocarbons that are formed when fat drips down onto the hot coals. With care you can avoid this problem.

Otherwise, any method that requires no additional fat or oil is fine; roasting, broiling and stewing are top-rated.

When sautéing or pan-broiling meat, use nonstick skillets. With these, only minimal oil, or perhaps no oil at all, will be necessary.

Do not baste meat or poultry with their own juices or butter. If basting is required, make up a marinade or sauce. You can do it by using a very small amount of vegetable oil to which you've added vinegar, lemon juice or wine to taste, as well as herbs, garlic and other seasonings. (A friend of mine suggests basting roast chicken with orange juice and pork with apple or pineapple juice.)

A trick for getting rid of some of the fat clinging to the surface of a pan-broiled or broiled steak or hamburger is to blot it with paper toweling just after cooking and before eating. Not very elegant, but effective.

One technique well worth mastering is that of skimming off fats from broths, pot roasts, braised meats, stews and sauces. In many recipes the fat in the meat melts off into the cooking liquid. But if the dish is allowed to sit for a minute before serving, the fat globules will rise to the top, where they can be spooned or skimmed off with a utensil made expressly for this purpose and called, appropriately enough, a skimmer. (You can find a skimmer in most dime stores, hardware stores and department stores.) When the heat is turned down very low, skimming can sometimes be done while the pot is still simmering on the burner.

An even better way to remove fat from a meat soup or stew is to place it in the refrigerator. Within a few hours the fat will rise to the top and solidify. Simply remove the hardened fat and discard.

33

What to Do about Cooking with Eggs

You know it already by now, but I'll say it one more time. Egg *yolks* are so high in cholesterol that unless you're an egg lover of the first degree, you should avoid them. One egg yolk contains in the neighborhood of 250 milligrams of cholesterol. Compare this to the 63 milligrams of cholesterol in a three-ounce serving of beef, lamb or pork, or the 27 milligrams of cholesterol in a glass of whole milk and you've got a better idea of the colossal cholesterol content of eggs.

It *is* possible to have an egg now and then and still eat a cancer-protective diet. Just remember that on those days when you eat an egg, you'll have to restrict other food of animal origin to stay within the recommended three hundred (or less) milligrams of cholesterol daily.

As for why eggs are included in some of the recipes that appear in this book, my assumption is that the food would be shared by several people, or that it would be eaten over several days. In either case, the one or two eggs in a recipe wouldn't be consumed by one person at one sitting.

Even so, it is preferable to experiment with egg substitutes or egg whites instead of whole eggs in these recipes. Egg whites as you know contain no cholesterol. (What do you do with the leftover yolk in such cases? How about giving it to a pet, or using it for plant food as the writers of *The Low Fat, Low Cholesterol Diet* suggest? One egg yolk mixed with a quart of water will feed ten plants at three ounces per pot.)

34

How to Choose Low-Risk Dairy Products

Keep in mind that milk products that say "low fat" on the label are slightly lower in fat than whole milk varieties, but not as low as skim milk products. "Low fat" products are usually made with a combination of whole and skim milk, or with partially skim milk. They are no substitute for skim milk products, but are an improvement over foods made with whole milk.

Unless you absolutely can't abide the taste, *skim* milk is preferable in your cereal, your coffee or tea and for drinking. (But remember, adults don't need great amounts of milk; water, sugar-free soda or fruit juice are better choices when you're just plain thirsty.)

Yogurt is a fine food. The yogurt cultures contain bacteria that may be useful in changing the ratio of anaerobic to aerobic bacteria in the colon to a more favorable one. Whenever possible choose yogurt made with skim milk. If this kind is unavailable at your local supermarket, consider making your own. It's easy to do and most good cookbooks include at least one yogurt recipe. (No, you don't need an electric yogurt maker; a crock or bowl will do just fine.)

I cannot emphasize enough the importance of careful label reading. Things are not always what they seem. For example, an imitation sour cream may not be made with cream, but it isn't necessarily fat-free either. Many of these products are made with hydrogenated oils or highly saturated vegetable oils such as coconut oil and have no place on the Anti-Cancer Diet.

35

How to Choose Cheese

Many cheeses have a high butterfat content, so it's important to use them with discretion. The bona fide cheese lover might prefer to eat more cheese and less meat and other high-fat foods. That's fine, so long as cholesterol levels are kept in mind. (See chapter 37, about trading off types of cholesterol.)

Skim milk cheeses—skim milk cottage cheese and skim milk ricotta—are entirely acceptable on an Anti-Cancer eating plan.

Less acceptable, but still okay within reason, are cheeses made with partially skim milk. They include Parmesan, sapsago, Edam and Gouda. Other cheeses that are sometimes made with partially skim milk are asiago, Gruyere, Limburger and mozzarella. If you buy prepackaged cheese, the label will tell you whether it's made with skim, whole, or partially skim milk. Otherwise, you have to rely on the knowledge of the person behind the counter. A knowledgeable cheese seller will be able to tell you which cheeses are made with what and perhaps introduce you to some of the less well-known cheeses from around the world that are made with skim or partially skim milk.

Most hard cheeses, unfortunately, are made with whole milk or whole milk and cream.

36

How to Make Your Own
Low-Fat Cottage Cheese

Cottage cheese with fresh chives or dill chopped into it or topped with luscious ripe strawberries or peaches makes a fine breakfast, lunch or snack. But do try to avoid creamed cottaged cheese, with its relatively high butterfat content.

If creamed cottage cheese is the only kind available, you can reduce the fat content by spooning it into a sieve and rinsing the cream and milk off the curds. Drain well before serving. (This little trick is a good idea even when you're using skim milk cottage cheese.)

37

How to Cut Down on Cholesterol

When pressed to make a choice, most people who are concerned about low-cholesterol, cancer-preventive eating (which is also good for heart health, let's not forget) would rather have meat several times a week and forgo eggs, cheese and other high-cholesterol foods. However, lately I've been meeting more and more men and women who are not particularly fond of meat. Given the choice, these people—perhaps you're one of them?—would prefer to do without some or all of the meat, poultry and fish on the Anti-Cancer Diet and eat an egg or cheese or more of something else instead.

The truth is, it doesn't matter how you cut down, as long as you keep cholesterol consumption at (or preferably below) three hundred milligrams per day. In other words, trading meat for an egg occasionally or even for good is perfectly okay. In effect, that's what the Seventh-day Adventists and other lacto-ovo-vegetarians have done.

Table 3 is designed to help you make these tradeoffs. It has four columns, numbered from 0 to 3. In the column numbered 0 are foods that are essentially cholesterol-free. (Of course, all fruits, cereals, vegetables, vegetable shortenings, margarine and nuts are cholesterol-free since they are nonanimal products. I have not

3. Keeping Cholesterol Consumption Down Through Tradeoffs

(100 mg. cholesterol)	(200 mg. cholesterol)	(300 mg. cholesterol)
1. Bakery Goods Angel food cake 2 slices bread of the kind made with egg substitutes, skim milk and vegetable shortening **2. Meat** None	**1. Bakery Goods** 3 oz. cake, pie, cookies or cornbread 2 doughnuts 1 sweet roll 1 brownie cookie 3 oz. egg noodles 2 pancakes **2. Meat** 4 oz. lean beef, veal, ham, lamb, turkey or chicken 2 oz. bacon	**1. Bakery Goods** May double amounts in "1" **2. Meat** May double amounts in "1" or use 5 oz. of less well-trimmed meats, or 4 oz. steak (marbled), pork chop, prime rib or hamburger	**1. Bakery Goods** 6 doughnuts 3 brownie cookies 6 pancakes **2. Meat** 2 oz. liver 6 oz. steak (marbled) 6 oz. pork chops 6 oz. prime rib 2 oz. sweetbreads ½ oz. calf brains 10 oz. turkey or chicken

3. *Fish*
None, but 2 oz. codfish, scallops or halibut nearly qualify

4. *Dairy Products*
Skim milk
Cottage cheese (low-fat or noncreamed)

5. *Eggs*
egg white (no yolk) egg substitutes

---

3. *Fish*
5 oz. codfish, trout or salmon
6 oz. scallops, halibut, codfish, tuna or clams
4 oz. haddock, perch, pike, mackerel or herring

4. *Dairy Products*
1 glass milk (8 oz.)
3 oz. (3 slices) cheese (Cheddar, American or Swiss)
6 oz. ice cream
12 oz. ice milk
4 pats butter
¼ cup cream

5. *Eggs*
None

---

3. *Fish*
4 oz. shrimp
5 oz. crab or lobster
6 oz. oysters

4. *Dairy Products*
May double amounts in "1" for cholesterol limits but total fat quantities will be unacceptable except with milk and cheese

5. *Eggs*
1 whole egg

---

3. *Fish*
6 oz. shrimp
8 oz. oysters
12 oz. haddock, perch, pike mackerel

4. *Dairy Products*
3 glasses whole milk
1 pint ice cream

5. *Eggs*
1½ eggs

listed them because they would play no part in a cholesterol tradeoff.)

The foods numbered 1 all have approximately one hundred milligrams of cholesterol in the amounts indicated. The weights given for meat and fish are uncooked weights; the weights given for baked goods are, of course, for the finished products.

The foods in the column numbered 2 have approximately 200 milligrams of cholesterol in the amounts indicated. You will note that some of the listings in this column are for the same foods in column "1," with allowances made for increased amounts. Also, I have listed an egg in this column, although at 250 milligrams of cholesterol per egg, this food really has a place about midway between column "2" and column "3."

In the column numbered 3 you will find foods that are especially high in cholesterol and larger quantities of some of the foods listed in columns "2" and "1." Calf brains, at three hundred milligrams of cholesterol per *half-ounce,* are higher than any other food in cholesterol content. I've included this item more as a curiosity than because I think anyone ought to eat a half-ounce portion of calf brains. Why bother?

Using the chart is relatively simple. If you want to restrict cholesterol intake to three hundred milligrams per day, you may have as much as you like of any foods in column "0" (though I hope you will also be guided by the need to stay within certain bounds with regard to calories of course). Or you could choose three of the items in column "1." Or one of the items in column "2" plus one of the items in column "1." Or, a single item from column "3."

Once again, vegetables, fruits and cereals can be used freely. Nuts need to be restricted only because of their high fat and calorie content.

38

How to Make Cereal a
Super Breakfast

Eggs at breakfast *are* nice and if you've been in the habit of having one (or two) each morning, you *will* miss them. But eggs, as you know, get a minus rating on the Anti-Cancer Diet, while cereals are a decided plus.

The trouble with cereal is that it can be so boring; a bowl of limp, soggy corn or wheat flakes isn't an especially exciting way to start the day. But the prospects can be improved considerably if you have on hand a supply of raisins and other dried fruits (apples, peaches, apricots, dates), chopped nuts, canned and fresh fruits, cinnamon and other spices, honey, brown sugar, jellies and preserves. With these to select from, you can make your own "cereal sundae"—a different one every morning if you like.

As you know, the best cereal choices are the ones made with whole grains. All bran, 40% bran flakes, and raisin bran are good. So are puffed wheat, granola, and rolled oats. Corn is a fine cereal grain but low on bulk.

Most of the presugared cereals are made with highly refined ingredients and are decidedly less desirable. Oatmeal is an excellent breakfast choice, though some people feel it's too much trouble because you have to cook it. (These same people usually don't object to cooking an egg.) If you haven't used oatmeal and some of the other cooked cereals for a while, give them another try. There's something very comforting and fortifying about starting the day with a hot cereal and you may find the extra time required makes very little difference to your morning schedule.

New on the scene (at least I've only recently become familiar with it) is granola. The kind you buy in the store has a nice taste and good nutrition, but the kind you make at home can be infinitely superior. Use the recipe on pages 246–247 to start with. Later you can vary it by adding different whole grains, fruits and nuts, and seeds. (Of course, you don't mix it fresh each morning. You make up a big batch and store it for later use in an air-tight container.)

Skim milk is always preferable to whole on cereals.

39

Now for Some Good Desserts

How do you end an Anti-Cancer meal? With icy cold watermelon in summer, baked banana with cinnamon and brown sugar in winter. With a walnut bar, an almond square, meringues, angelfood cake. Fresh strawberries topped with kirsch, mandarin orange slices with nuts and honey. Oatmeal raisin cookies, Italian ices, extravagant gelatin concoctions, fresh fruit cocktail topped with yogurt and dates, rhubarb sherbet, cherry almond whip. The list could go on and on.

A host of good tasting and acceptable desserts are included in the meal-planning section. With a little imagination I'm sure you'll be able to come up with many more of your own.

Stay away from ice cream or use it as a tradeoff according to Table 3 in chapter 37. Its butterfat content is high. Ice milk is better but not much. Sherbets and Italian ices are much better.

Most cakes are out because they're made with butter or solid shortening and eggs. But angelfood cake and any other recipe you run across that can be made without eggs (or with egg substitutes) and with no or a minimal amount of vegetable oil will do very nicely. In short, the same rules apply in the dessert category as in any other: no fat or very small amounts of fat, with liquid vege-

table oil or other unsaturated fat taking precedence over saturated **fats** of animal origin.

One all-time dessert favorite (and unfortunately a snack favorite as well), chocolate, doesn't appear on my list because of its high fat and sugar content. I like chocolate in almost any form—drinks, candy, ice milk, the works. Unfortunately, logic requires that its use be restricted.

Chocolate is 50 percent fat by weight, and since there are nine calories per gram in fat (compared to four calories in a gram of carbohydrate or protein), this means that about three-fourths of the calories in chocolate come from fat. Yes, it's vegetable fat, so there is no cholesterol, but most of the fat in chocolate is the saturated kind. It must be severely restricted or eliminated from the Anti-Cancer Diet. Carob can be used in many recipes as a substitute for chocolate; it is relatively low in fat and is derived from the locust tree. (In Biblical times it was called St. John's bread.)

Sugar, as we have indicated, is not linked to any kind of cancer, but in the interest of keeping total calorie consumption within reasonable bounds, more than one serving of dessert is not advised.

40

How to Snack Safely

There's very little point in modifying your meals along cancer-protective lines if you don't change your snacking habits as well.

As you might expect, potato chips, corn chips, taco chips and other chips, as well as commercially baked cake, pie and cookies are all unacceptable because of their very high fat content. The same is true of ice cream. In the case of baked goods eggs and chocolate are used liberally in their preparation. If this sounds as though there's nothing left to snack on, think again.

Fresh raw fruits and vegetables are ideal. (Chilled raw cauliflower, perhaps with a little salt, is a real treat, as are many other chilled raw vegetables.) Dried fruits are excellent. Skim milk yogurt topped with fruit or a tablespoon or so of jelly or jam stirred in is also good. A slice of whole grain bread spread with jelly satisfies a sweet tooth. A serving of sherbet or Italian ice is refreshing in summer. Even a fruit-flavor popsicle is fine. Try a few rye wafers, wheat wafers, bread sticks or melba toast. Any of these with crushed sardines, well drained of oil, spread on top makes a good-tasting snack.

An *occasional* handful of nuts is okay. Occasional is the key word; because of their high fat content nuts should only be eaten once in a while.

41

How to Eat Better by
Reading Labels

Taken together, a lot of small changes can add up to a very big difference. The changes I'm talking about can be effected merely by reading the labels of everything you buy at the supermarket, comparing different varieties or brands and purchasing the one that scores highest for cancer-protective ingredients (or lowest for objectionable ingredients).

Keep in mind the general principle that on labels and packages the first ingredient will be the principal one; the last ingredient will be present in the smallest quantity. Thus, it's pretty safe to assume that if the label of brand X mentions fat as a second-place ingredient whereas fat appears in fourth or fifth place on the label of brand Y, brand Y is the better choice.

If possible, then, try to avoid products that have a fat or an oil, eggs or cream high up in their list of ingredients.

Unless you really need the extra calories, seek out canned fruits packed in water or light syrup rather than heavy syrup. Some canned fish is also packed in water, and these too are preferable.

Breads and cereals made with whole grains are more desirable than the highly refined products, and nowadays the food companies usually make a point of specifying that their products are whole grain on the label.

The product made with skim milk or skim milk solids is always preferable to the one made with whole milk. If whole milk is used, the farther down on the list of ingredients, the better.

42

How to Get Your Children off to a Good Start

Most fathers and mothers believe that feeding their children properly is one of their primary responsibilities. And indeed it is. A good diet during childhood is even more important than ever now that we have evidence that overnourishment in the early years may impose additional cancer risks (particularly of breast cancer).

We can, then, do our children an enormous favor by seeing to it that they eat well right from the very beginning. That means skim milk instead of whole milk from the age of two on. (As I mentioned earlier, some pediatricians recommend that babies go directly from infant formula or breast to skim milk in a bottle or cup.) It also means corn oil margarine instead of butter, more whole grain cereals instead of the refined presweetened kind and so on right down the line. In other words, the Anti-Cancer Diet that helps protect adults from malignancy is equally valuable, if not more so for children.

As a father, I know that children can be finicky. Part of the key to helping them eat well is to *listen* to them. For example, if a child says that he or she can't stand the taste of a particular cooked vegetable, don't force the issue. Instead, offer the vegetable raw. Sometimes a child who won't go near cooked green beans, cauliflower, spinach, cabbage or carrots relishes the crisp, crunchy texture of these same vegetables uncooked. When you're preparing vegetables, put a few pieces aside to serve raw to the finicky child. Trust your child's appetite. Children won't starve themselves to death. They *will* eat and they do. But they usually have the good sense to wait until they're hungry. What bothers many parents is that their children's hunger often doesn't coincide with family mealtimes. If this is the case at your house, what can you do about it?

You *could* place severe restrictions on snacks so that by the time suppertime rolls around the kids will be ravenous. The trouble with this approach is that a hungry child is usually a cranky, utterly disagreeable person to have around and in the long run it may not be worth the effort to hold out. A better way is to have good healthy snacks around the house at all times. Things like skim milk yogurt, fresh fruits and vegetables, dried fruits, sliced chicken or turkey, well-drained tuna fish. Keep them where the children can serve themselves and tell them that they're allowed to do so. And remember that a carrot served at mealtime is no more nutritious than a carrot eaten an hour before. The difference is mainly in the mind of the cook.

If you want the children's company at mealtimes, by all means have them join you. But don't worry if they don't clean their plates. With healthy snacks they don't need to. Mealtime battle scenes don't help anyone's digestion, and when children are very young, good nutrition is more important than having them eat on schedule. (Of course, in this approach, if the snacks are junk food, your children's nutrition *will* suffer.)

As children get older, they usually settle into more grown-up eating schedules. But another problem may crop up because now they're spending more time in their friends' homes where they may be given undesirable food to snack on. Fortunately, by this age your child is probably old enough to listen to and understand your reasons for not keeping potato chips and ice cream around the house. He or she may not be entirely happy about the situation, but it's better to explain than to appear stubborn and arbitrary.

In the end, you can't control what an older child eats away from home. But you'll have the satisfaction of knowing that you've gotten him or her off to a good start. That counts for *something*. And with any luck, Anti-Cancer eating habits begun early in life will help shape your children's adult eating habits for the better.

43

Entertaining on the Anti-Cancer Diet

On festive occasions people who are normally watchful about what they eat always tend to put aside their everyday food concerns "for the sake of the guests." Going overboard once in a while, serving creamed soups, heavy sauces, rich desserts and the like, isn't catastrophic. (The truth is, even if you ate along Anti-Cancer lines only part of the time, your diet would still be superior to that of most Americans.)

But you don't have to deviate on special occasions. Lean meat, poultry or fish, fresh, perfectly prepared vegetables, luscious ripe fruits—these are foods worthy of anyone or any occasion.

If you doubt it, think of roast beef, parsley potatoes and a crisp spinach salad accompanied by a fine red wine and followed by a bowl of scarlet apples, purple and green grapes. Or roast chicken garnished with lemon slices and served with broiled peaches, wild rice, endive and raw mushroom salad, a mellow rosé wine and angelfood cake for dessert. Why turn away from such fare?

True, when cooking for company you may want to give additional thought to the "extras," take special pains with a soup stock, make an effort to find fresh herbs for seasoning, search out the most attractive blemish-free fruits and vegetables, add a touch of wine to a recipe, bake a special bread, use imaginative garnishes.

You may also want to make some concessions to your guests: butter on the table and a gravy or sauce for their meat; two salad dressings, lemon and herbs for you, a conventional cheese or oil dressing for them. You needn't go much further than that.

What if they notice that you've chosen to eat one way while they're eating another? What if they ask why? You could mumble something about being on a diet, but why not explain instead? It could lead to some lively after-dinner conversation. And who knows? They might decide to try cancer-protective eating themselves.

44

How to Eat Out and Eat Safe

Even though you have limited control over what you eat when you eat out, you can still be guided by a few of the Anti-Cancer principles.

Common sense dictates how: in a restaurant, order fish, poultry, or veal, broiled or baked, and tell the waiter to hold the gravy or sauce. Broiled or roast beef, pork or lamb are okay too. Just remember to trim off visible fat before eating. Steamed vegetables, as always, are best. If the menu indicates that vegetables are served with hollandaise or other sauce, ask the waiter to bring yours without. Clear broths and consommés are a better choice than creamed soups. Salad should be served with dressing on the side so that you can pour on as much (or as little) as you want. Better still, ask for a lemon wedge. For dessert, fresh fruit, melon or sherbet.

Don't be afraid to specify what you want. Ask for whole wheat bread. Ask for margarine instead of butter. Ask for milk or skim milk instead of cream for your coffee.

As a guest in someone's house your options are more limited. But you can pass up butter, sauces and gravies and trim all the fat from your meat. Even these small changes make a difference.

45

How to Modify Standard Recipes
to Fit the Anti-Cancer Diet

Cooking is a creative art, not an exact science. Very few recipes are so precisely planned that there is no leeway for substituting one kind of ingredient for another. In the Anti-Cancer Diet the idea is to substitute low- (or lower-) risk ingredients for high-risk ingredients. The following list will give you an idea of what kind of substitutions you can make. (You will probably be able to come up with some interesting variations of your own. If so, I'd like to know about them.)

Skim milk can be substituted for whole milk or cream in almost any recipe. (The obvious exception is a recipe that calls for cream for whipping.)

Corn oil margarine can be substituted for butter under almost all circumstances.

Liquid vegetable oil can be substituted for margarine, butter or solid shortenings in many recipes, though not usually in breads, cakes or pastries.

Lemon or some other fruit juice can substitute for rich sauces, gravies or dressings.

Cruciferous vegetables (broccoli, Brussels sprouts, cabbage, cauliflower and spinach) can replace other vegetables in soups, stews, salads and other recipes calling for vegetables.

Many recipes calling for eggs will be equally good if egg whites only or egg substitutes are used instead. (In general, plan to use two egg whites for every whole egg called for in a recipe.)

Happy cooking!

PART III

MEAL PLANS AND RECIPES

46

How Meal Plans and Recipes
Can Help You Follow the
Anti-Cancer Diet

The menus and recipes in this section are included mainly to give you an idea of how delightfully easy and enjoyable it can be to stay on an Anti-Cancer food regimen. You can follow the meal planner to the letter (there are ten days' worth of spring-summer menus and ten days' worth of fall/winter menus with appropriate recipes for each.) Or, you may prefer to use the planner for reference only as a guide from which to model your own food plans.

As you glance through the menus and recipes you will see that most of the dishes are old familiar favorites, somewhat modified so they're made with less fat or oil, or with more bulk or roughage than the traditional versions you may have been serving and eating for years. Other dishes may be new to you. I hope you'll try them—for variety and because they're made with ingredients that are especially desirable on an Anti-Cancer food plan—but it's not absolutely necessary that you do.

The Anti-Cancer Diet does not depend on any one food or group of foods (any food plan that does so is almost by definition "faddish," and also probably ultimately unhealthy). Instead, it's based on a collection of principles: less fat, less cholesterol, plenty of protein but from a wider variety of sources (including fish and vegetable protein) than you may be accustomed to, more bulk, fewer calories.

So far I haven't stressed the desirability of cutting back on calories. Here's why: if you follow the other suggestions, consuming less fat and oil and at the same time not going overboard on sweets and highly refined carbohydrates, a calorie reduction will occur almost automatically. (And because you'll also be eating substantial amounts of fruits and vegetables and significantly more satisfying high-bulk foods, you won't feel at all as though you're on a diet.) However, just to refresh your memory as to *why* calories count on an Anti-Cancer regimen, remember that in almost all test situations animals that were underfed developed far fewer tumors on exposure to carcinogens than overfed animals.

The average daily calorie intake in this country is approximately thirty-four hundred. In Japan it is only two thousand. Even taking into account that the average Japanese needs fewer calories because he or she is smaller in stature than the average American, these figures are still dramatic testimony as to why obesity and obesity-related ailments are so common in this country. When you also consider that fully 42 percent of our calories come in the form of fat or oil, as opposed to 13 percent in the Japanese diet, you can see why the cancers of overnutrition are so prevalent here but relatively rare in Japan.

The fact is, we would probably all benefit by cutting our calorie consumption in half. That would give us an average daily caloric intake of seventeen hundred. You can get perfectly adequate amounts of all the essential nutrients on seventeen hundred calories a day, and the cancer-protective aspect of such a regimen could be enormous. However, desirable though seventeen hundred calories a day might be for most people, I'm not going to come down hard on this point. The attempt might be psychologically defeating to some who, discovering that they don't feel comfortable living on seventeen hundred calories a day, may become discouraged and give up on the Anti-Cancer Diet entirely. I wouldn't want that to happen, so I want to assure you that you'll be way ahead in terms of cancer protection (and reduce your likelihood of developing many other diseases as well) merely by staying within the guidelines suggested throughout this book. That means that within these guidelines you can have reasonable amounts of meat and other foods of animal origin, and (with a few obvious exceptions such as bread, pasta, noodles) probably as much as you want of everything else. What could be easier?

Following are a group of Anti-Cancer meal plans for spring and summer and another group for fall and winter. Recipes for all dishes that are starred (*) are given following the section of meal plans and are listed in alphabetical order.

47

Bread: Should You or Shouldn't You

Bread is optional in the menus that follow. In other words, if you're one of those people for whom a meal simply isn't satisfying without bread, have some. Choose mostly whole grain breads, for their fiber content and because they're generally nutritionally superior. Also, look for breads that are made with liquid vegetable oils rather than solid or hydrogenated (saturated) shortening. Keep in mind that when a label merely says "shortening" (without indicating what kind) it usually means that hydrogenated (saturated) fat has been used. If you buy at a bakery where the bread is unlabeled, remember that rolls and buns are usually made with solid shortening and probably contain eggs.

If you've got a weight problem and/or eat bread only out of habit without being particularly fond of it, why not pass it up entirely, or at least eat less of it? Have one slice if you used to have two. Try open-faced sandwiches, which automatically cut your bread consumption in half—assuming you don't eat twice as many sandwiches.

As for what you put on bread, corn oil margarine is a better choice than butter (the fat content is the same, but butter is high in cholesterol). For an Anti-Cancer diet, jelly or jam is better than either. And *no* spread is best. The different whole grain breads with their various rich, nutlike flavors, as well as French or Italian bread, crusty on the outside and chewy inside, taste so good by themselves that they don't really need a spread to make them better.

48

Meal Plans for Spring and Summer

PLAN #1

One of the best things about spring and summer is the abundance of fresh fruits and vegetables. The possibilities are endless, and you can be adventurous. Get a good cookbook on vegetarian cooking and look for recipes that contain no cream, butter or oil, and only small amounts of vegetable oil, margarine or skim milk cheeses. Cut down on these ingredients whenever possible. For example, steam vegetables instead of sautéing.

Breakfast

    whole fresh strawberries with sugar
  *granola with skim milk
    whole wheat toast
    beverage

Lunch

    pineapple juice
    sliced turkey (white meat) with raw spinach on pumpernickel
      bread
    sliced tomato
    whole plum
    beverage

Supper

> chicken consommé
> *fish and rice salad
> steamed green beans marinated with lemon juice and served
> > cold, on lettuce
> *rhubarb-strawberry sherbet
> beverage

PLAN #2

Skim milk yogurt is an especially valuable food–nutritious, low in fat and a valuable source of protein and "friendly" bacteria. It's easy to make. Use it often, mixing with any fruit in season and toppings of your choice—raisins, cinnamon, honey, dried fruits, nuts, granola. Add to salads and salad dressings, and to cooked vegetables.

Breakfast

> prune juice
> *French toast with sliced peaches
> beverage

Lunch

> skim milk yogurt with chopped dates, cantaloupe chunks and
> > honey
> celery sticks
> cracked wheat bread
> beverage

Supper

> chilled pineapple tidbits
> *pepper steak
> boiled rice
> salad: chicory, raw spinach, cold slightly cooked broccoli,
> > sliced raw cauliflower and tomatoes with lemon juice
> *lemon ice
> beverage

PLAN #3

Read labels of the many canned fish products available in supermarkets. Look for tuna, salmon and sardines packed in water, no-oil sauces or soya or cottonseed oil rather than olive oil (olive oil is more saturated than most vegetable oils). Drain carefully if packed in oil, or better yet, rinse off the oils before using the fish.

Breakfast

>   broiled grapefruit (sprinkle ½ grapefruit with brown sugar or
>   honey and dash of cinnamon; broil until slightly brown)
>   shredded wheat with chopped dried apricots, skim milk
>   soya toast
>   beverage

Lunch

>   small can salmon on lettuce or spinach leaves
>   carrot sticks and raw cauliflower flowerets
>   whole wheat bread
>   mandarin oranges with raisins
>   beverage

Supper

>   apple juice
>   *veal cutlets with Marsala
>   *molded tomato salad
>   peas
>   *oatmeal-raisin cookies
>   beverage

PLAN #4

Tabouli is an "exotic" treat, especially if you have fresh mint and parsley. It is usually served on lettuce leaves but can also be used to fill the round, flat Syrian pita bread. You don't have to be a perfectionist about the ingredients in tabouli, but you should try it once exactly as the recipe specifies. After you know what a classic tabouli is, you can try your own combinations of vegetables and herbs. Keep it crunchy and very fresh.

Breakfast

   banana shake (spin in blender 1 whole banana, 1 cup skim
      milk, ½ tsp. vanilla, ½ tsp. sugar)
   oatmeal toast
   beverage

Lunch

   *tabouli (Lebanese salad) in pita bread
   skim milk yogurt with cherries
   beverage

Supper

   cranberry juice
   *pot au feu (French beef and vegetable supper soup)
   salad: shredded romaine and green pepper strips with lemon
      juice
   sliced oranges with nuts and honey
   beverage

PLAN #5

   A nicely trimmed fresh artichoke makes any meal more special.
The yogurt, served as a dip for the artichoke leaves, provides the
protein in this meal. Experiment with herbs and seasonings to
make a dip you like. Artichokes in season are a good buy and a
good source of vitamins.

Breakfast

   tangerine
   bran cereal with skim milk, honey and raisins
   *blueberry muffin
   beverage

Lunch

   *artichokes with yogurt
   tomato wedges
   oatmeal bread
   beverage

Supper

chicken consommé with minced celery

*tuna casserole

salad: raw spinach, lettuce, sliced celery, chopped tomato, chopped scallions and lemon juice

cherry-almond whip (whip slightly firm cherry gelatin, add chopped cherries and almonds, 1–2 tbs. rum or ½ tsp. rum flavoring, and chill; serve with grated almonds and whole cherry)

beverage

PLAN #6

Most breakfasts include a cereal or bread. But why not try something different? Have you ever had soup for breakfast? Leftover cold fish or meat? For some people, such breakfasts are a treat. (They're economical, too, since leftovers are used.)

The lamb roast, of course, must be trimmed carefully before cooking and trimmed of fat before eating, too.

Breakfast

½ grapefruit

fish on toasted English muffin (mash sardines, salmon or leftover fish with lemon juice, chopped mushrooms, minced onion, fennel and pepper; spread on muffin and broil until bubbly)

beverage

Lunch

*onion-tomato soup

celery and carrot sticks

French bread

sliced whole peach with skim milk ricotta cheese, honey and raisins

beverage

Supper

vegetable juice

roast leg of lamb

French-style peas (cook 2–3 cups shredded lettuce, 1 thinly
sliced onion, and 2 cups fresh or frozen peas in 2 tbs.
margarine, covered, stirring often; season to taste)
baked potato
crushed pineapple in lime gelatin, with skim milk yogurt and
honey topping
beverage

PLAN #7

The luncheon salad included in this plan is another recipe that
hardly needs to be written out. Try it anyway, and next time use
your imagination to mix up your own.

Breakfast

apple juice
skim milk cottage cheese with chopped dates
oatmeal toast with *cinnamon sugar
beverage

Lunch

*fruit and vegetable salad on lettuce
whole wheat bread
beverage

Supper

tomato juice
*pan-broiled fillet of sole
steamed Brussels sprouts with lemon juice
boiled new potatoes (cook in skin 20–40 minutes in salted
water, roll in small amount of margarine and chopped
parsley)
*frozen lemon dessert
beverage

PLAN #8

Fish chowder is tasty and nutritious. Once you know the basic
procedure, you can use any variety of fish and vegetables. It's hard

to go wrong with this one. The flavor is hardly ever exactly the same as last time, but it is always good.

Breakfast

> orange juice
> *rolled oat cereal with grated apple
> beverage

Lunch

> English muffin, topped with slice Canadian bacon, pineapple slice, broiled slowly
> cold marinated steamed Brussels sprouts
> whole orange
> beverage

Supper

> cranberry juice
> *vegetable-fish chowder
> salad: lettuce, sliced celery, tomatoes, green pepper strips, lemon juice
> French bread
> fresh raspberries

PLAN #9

When making pasta, look for the ripest (vine-ripened) tomatoes. Home-grown would be ideal. Or if you've found a brand of canned tomatoes that you think is really tasty, you might use it instead. When the tomatoes are good, this is a very special dish.

Breakfast

> sliced fresh pineapple
> dark bread with peanut butter, 1 tbs. honey drizzled over top
> beverage

Lunch

> *carrot-apple salad
> skim milk cottage cheese

whole banana
beverage

Supper

grapefruit juice
*pasta with fresh tomatoes
salad: lettuce, raw spinach, sliced raw mushrooms, watercress, chopped raw cauliflower with lemon juice
Italian bread
green grapes

PLAN #10

Cheeses should be used infrequently and sparingly, and it does
matter which ones you use. Some are made from partly skim
milk—Swiss,. Jarlsberg, Edam, Parmesan and sapsago. Others are
either whole milk or skim milk based. Choose the skim milk varieties (cottage cheese, mozzarella, ricotta). If you shop at a specialty cheese store, ask the salesperson about skim milk cheeses;
there are many more than you'd find in the ordinary supermarket.

Breakfast

fresh blueberries and sliced peaches with skim milk yogurt
cracked wheat toast
beverage

Lunch

broiled cheese sandwich (place a slice of Swiss or Jarlsberg
on rye bread, sprinkle with minced pimiento, broil
quickly)
whole peach
beverage

Supper

apple juice
broiled sirloin
sliced tomatoes with chopped basil and scallions
steamed cauliflower with lemon juice
watermelon
beverage

PLAN #11

Meringues add a special touch to a dessert of fresh or frozen berries or other summer fruits. They're easy and fun to make (children like to shape them) and can be made ahead of time.

Breakfast

> cantaloupe
> shredded wheat, skim milk, honey
> whole wheat toast
> beverage

Lunch

> skim milk cottage cheese with chives
> sliced tomato
> pumpernickel bread
> whole orange

Supper

> tomato juice
> *chicken sauté
> steamed broccoli with lemon juice
> salad: lettuce, romaine, chopped celery, cooked sliced beets,
>   lemon juice
> *meringues with fresh strawberries and sugar
> beverage

PLAN #12

Skim milk ricotta tastes something like cottage cheese (perhaps a little smoother and milder). It's delicious mixed with sliced fresh peaches or apples and a little cinnamon.

Breakfast

> ½ cantaloupe
> skim milk ricotta with sliced fresh peach and dash of cin-
>   namon
> beverage

Lunch

chilled marinated broccoli (steamed) on lettuce
slice of Edam cheese
whole wheat bread
whole plum
beverage

Supper

tomato juice
broiled swordfish (brush swordfish steak or any fish steak
with scant amount of oil; salt and pepper and broil 2–3
inches from flame until fish flakes easily; garnish with
lemon slice or wedge and parsley)
boiled potatoes, rolled in small amount margarine and
chopped parsley
salad: dill, green pepper, raw mushrooms, romaine, scallions
*angelfood cake with raspberries
beverage

PLAN #13

Fruit salad is one dish that pleases almost everyone. The fruit
has to be ripe but it doesn't have to be beautiful. This is a good
way to use bruised pieces. If you're lucky enough to have juicy,
ripe fruit, you won't have to add sweetener or juice. If you want
sweeter fruit salad add apple or orange juice. If you are making it
ahead of time and including apples or bananas, add lemon juice to
prevent discoloring.

Breakfast

orange juice
skim milk ricotta with sliced apple, cinnamon and granola
whole wheat toast
beverage

Lunch

fruit salad: fresh cantaloupe, peaches, banana, blueberries
and orange with nuts
slice of Swiss cheese

oatmeal bread
beverage

Supper

tomato juice
broiled pork chops
corn on the cob
*cole slaw
watermelon
beverage

PLAN #14

Children especially enjoy "milk shakes" for breakfast. There are
many ways to add nutrition and flavor to a blender shake. To
make sure it's really icy cold on a hot summer morning, add
crushed ice to the mixture before blending. You can use frozen
fruit that is partially thawed.

Breakfast

peach blender shake (fresh peach and skim milk mixed in
    blender; sugar rarely necessary)
toasted raisin bread

Lunch

tuna plate: tuna on raw spinach leaves with sliced tomato,
    green pepper
rye crackers
whole peach
beverage

Supper

chopped apple and lemon juice
*veal with mushrooms
steamed Brussels sprouts with lemon juice
fresh pepper salad (thinly sliced red pepper, green pepper,
    onion, marinated one hour or more in 2 tbs. cider vinegar,
    2 tbs. water, 1 tsp. salt, ¼ tsp. pepper, 1 tbs. sugar; drain
    before serving)
fresh blueberries
beverage

PLAN #15

Pizza doesn't have to be complicated. When fresh tomatoes are available, you can make pizza in minutes, with no sauce. Try your own favorite toppings—chopped onions, green peppers, mushrooms, etc.

Breakfast

> fresh blueberries and skim milk cottage cheese
> *oatmeal-applesauce bread
> beverage

Lunch

> easy fresh pizza (on half English muffin, place layer of sliced skim milk mozzarella, sliced tomato, sprinkle of garlic salt, pepper, oregano, grated Parmesan cheese; bake in hot oven 10–15 minutes)
> cucumber spears
> cantaloupe
> beverage

Supper

> tomato juice
> *pork and zucchini casserole
> salad: cold slightly steamed cauliflower, chopped sweet red pepper, lettuce and watercress with lemon juice
> pineapple gelatin whip (lemon gelatin prepared with juice from canned pineapple, partially set, whipped and mixed with crushed pineapple and chopped nuts)
> beverage

PLAN #16

Everyone should learn how to make gazpacho. When summer vegetables are at their peak, this soup, chilled well, is tasty and refreshing. It's easy, too—no cooking!

The salmon hash recipe can be found in many cookbooks; here we have just eliminated the egg yolk and used egg white to bind the ingredients.

Breakfast

> whole nectarine
> wild rice cooked and served cold as cereal with skim milk,
>   sugar or honey, and raisins
> whole wheat toast
> beverage

Lunch

> *gazpacho
> Italian bread with slice of Swiss cheese and raw spinach leaf
> cantaloupe
> beverage

Supper

> grapefruit juice
> *salmon hash
> steamed broccoli with lemon juice
> sliced peaches with blueberries
> beverage

PLAN #17

Fresh dill has a flavor all its own. Try it in these dilled brown muffins. It can also be chopped and added to tossed green salads and sprinkled on many vegetables—it's especially good with cauliflower, green beans and cucumbers. It is nutritionally valuable and one of the cancer-protective vegetables to be added to the diet as often as possible.

Breakfast

> honeydew melon
> granola, skim milk, raisins
> whole wheat toast
> beverage

Lunch

> cottage cheese with sliced radishes, celery, green pepper, salt
>   and pepper
> *dilled brown muffin

whole nectarine
beverage

Supper

pineapple juice
broiled lamb chops
broiled tomatoes (sprinkle thick slices of ripe tomatoes with
salt and pepper, basil; broil until slightly browned)
thinly sliced green pepper and red onion on raw spinach
leaves with lemon juice
pineapple cubes and strawberries with mint and powdered
sugar
beverage

PLAN #18

This supper can be made ahead and can save you a little work
on the following day. Cook an extra chicken when preparing
chicken-in-a-pot. Remove meat from bones and refrigerate to use
next day as chicken salad or sliced in a sandwich. Or make
chicken pot pie.

Breakfast

sliced oranges with skim milk yogurt and brown sugar
cracked wheat toast
beverage

Lunch

vegetable salad (chopped raw cauliflower and raw mushrooms, shredded carrots, minced onion, salt, sugar and
lemon juice) on raw spinach leaves
*bran muffin
nectarine
beverage

Supper

apple juice
*chicken-in-a-pot
rice with peas
tomato relish salad (chopped or diced ripe tomatoes, cucum-

bers, green peppers, scallions, radishes and parsley, tossed
with lemon juice, salt and pepper and fresh or dried basil)
fresh cherries, pitted, and cubed fresh cantaloupe
beverage

PLAN #19

Whipping gelatin before it is firm makes the final product look a
little more festive. Combining the whipped gelatin with fresh fruits
adds texture and interest. Add your own favorite extras—nuts,
granola, etc.

Breakfast

chilled fresh pineapple chunks, mint garnish
toasted raisin bread topped with mixture of skim milk cottage
cheese, brown sugar and cinnamon and broiled 2 minutes
beverage

Lunch

chicken salad: chopped chicken with diced celery and apples, moistened with skim milk yogurt and honey, on lettuce
pumpernickel bread
beverage

Supper

vegetable juice with lemon wedge
*cod Provençale
steamed cauliflower with lemon juice
sliced cucumber and green pepper
raspberry gelatin, whipped, topped with fresh raspberries
beverage

PLAN #20

This supper is a meal to cook on one of the cooler summer
days. Or if there is no such thing as a cool summer day where you
live, roast the meat in the evening and serve cold the next day. Or
roast early in the day when no one is home and you can be out of
the kitchen while the oven is on.

Breakfast

  sliced peach
  whole grain cereal with skim milk
  beverage

Lunch

  *cauliflower soup
  celery and carrot sticks
  whole wheat bread
  cherries
  beverage

Supper

  tomato juice
  roast beef
  *mushroom-zucchini salad
  *potato salad
  fresh strawberries (with 1 tbs. kirsch, if desired)

PLAN #21

In ratatouille, the tomatoes in particular must be ripe and tasty. (It's better to use good canned plum tomatoes than bland hothouse fresh ones.) When you have good sun-ripened vegetables and cook this dish with a light hand, taking care not to overcook, the result is something special. The several vegetables should each be recognizable.

Breakfast

  fresh fruit salad with granola topping
  *oatmeal-applesauce bread
  beverage

Lunch

  sliced roast beef and lettuce
  cold marinated diced cauliflower and chopped red pepper
  whole plum
  beverage

Supper

grapes
*ratatouille
salad: Boston lettuce, raw spinach, sliced celery and scallions, chopped pimiento, sliced fresh mushrooms and lemon juice
French bread
cantaloupe
beverage

49

Meal Plans for Fall and Winter

PLAN #1

Poaching fish is easy, nearly foolproof. By varying the ingredients in the poaching liquid (different herbs, wines, chopped vegetables) you'll find your own favorite combinations.

For lunch you may prefer to chop the vegetables fine and spread the mixture on pumpernickel toast.

Breakfast

whole tangerine
*whole wheat pancakes
beverage

Lunch

vegetable and cottage cheese salad on lettuce (2 cups skim milk cottage cheese mixed with up to 2 cups of any combination of thinly sliced radishes, celery, and scallions; salt and pepper to taste)
canned plums
beverage

Supper

vegetable juice
*poached fish
steamed turnip cubes, with lemon juice, nutmeg and brown
    sugar or honey
salad: medium-sized pieces of cucumber, green pepper, and
    shredded raw cabbage, with fresh lime juice
whole sliced fresh pear with skim milk yogurt–honey topping
beverage

PLAN #2

The aroma of pork roast in the oven and apples and onions
sautéing on the stove almost makes the cold weather worth it. Be
very careful about trimming off all fat before roasting the meat,
and use a bare minimum of margarine in preparing the apple and
onion dish. Note that there is very little other animal fat in the rest
of this day's menu.

Breakfast

pineapple juice
cooked whole wheat cereal with wheat germ, brown sugar,
    chopped walnuts
beverage

Lunch

tuna plate: plain tuna, cherry tomatoes, sliced cucumbers,
    sliced green peppers, on lettuce and raw spinach leaves
whole wheat bread
whole orange
beverage

Dinner

consommé
pork roast
*onions and apples
steamed spinach, with lemon juice, nutmeg and seasonings to
    taste
quick-glazed pineapple slices with nuts (dip slices in brown

sugar, broil, top with chopped walnuts)
beverage

PLAN #3

Spinach is a good source of vitamins A and C and is one of the cruciferous vegetables. Use it often raw as a salad ingredient and on sandwiches—in fact, anywhere you might have used lettuce leaves in the past. There are persons who form kidney stones of a particular type who must avoid spinach. If you have had kidney stones, your doctor may restrict your intake of this vegetable.

Breakfast

orange juice
shredded wheat with sliced banana, skim milk
whole wheat toast
beverage

Lunch

cottage cheese and pineapple chunks on lettuce or raw spinach
toasted oatmeal bread with *cinnamon sugar
whole apple
beverage

Supper

pear nectar
*veal roast with vegetables
salad: raw spinach, romaine, chopped scallions, green pepper, with lemon juice
*dinner rolls
orange gelatin with whole pitted cherries (prepare gelatin with cherry juice from can instead of water; cube gelatin and mix with whole cherries)
beverage

PLAN #4

Corned beef is not recommended on the Anti-Cancer Diet, but if you include in the meal many sources of vitamin C, you can get away with it. Remember that the vitamin has to be present at the same meal to be effective, and it is our suggestion it be in food rather than tablets.

Breakfast

> whole orange
> dry whole grain cereal with skim milk, raisins, honey
> English muffin
> beverage

Lunch

> chicken consommé with rice, chopped onion, celery, pimiento
> skim milk yogurt with fruit of choice
> whole wheat bread
> beverage

Supper

> tomato juice
> *corned beef and cabbage
> salad: sliced celery, radishes, green peppers and spinach with
>   lemon juice
> canned plums
> beverage

PLAN #5

The leftover corned beef is from the previous day's supper.

Breakfast

> grapefruit juice
> hot oatmeal with brown sugar
> *bran muffins
> beverage

Lunch

> corned beef and spinach leaf on rye bread with mustard
> dill pickles
> whole fresh orange
> beverage

Supper

    *kedgeree (fish and rice with curry)
    steamed broccoli with lemon juice
    shredded lettuce and grated carrot with lemon juice
    fresh or canned pear slices with powdered sugar and cin-
       namon
    beverage

PLAN #6

Cauliflower is another cruciferous vegetable that can be used in many ways. Break it into flowerets or slice and eat as a finger food. It can be coarsely chopped for salads or minced fine to add a crunchy texture to other cooked vegetables (much as you might use nuts for texture).

Breakfast

    whole pear
    *nut waffles
    beverage

Lunch

    skim milk yogurt with orange sections
    whole wheat toast with peanut butter and chopped apples
    beverage

Supper

    grapefruit juice
    roast chicken
    *acorn squash
    salad: lettuce, sliced raw cauliflower, scallions, raw mush-
       rooms, dill, with lemon juice
    *walnut bars
    beverage

PLAN #7

Whenever you cook soybeans, prepare more than you need for your recipe and set the extra beans aside in the refrigerator to toss into salads.

If you haven't discovered homemade granola yet, you're in for a treat. Experiment with combinations until you find just the blend you like. The essential element is the whole grain cereal.

Breakfast

    apricot nectar
    *granola with skim milk yogurt and nutmeg
    oatmeal bread
    beverage

Lunch

    sliced chicken
    salad: lettuce, scallions, cherry tomato, sliced raw cauliflower
    *walnut bars
    beverage

Supper

    tangerine sections
    *soybean-mushroom dish
    cooked macaroni with margarine, salt and pepper
    sliced cucumber, green pepper rings, chopped parsley and
        pimiento on lettuce
    frozen strawberries
    beverage

PLAN #8

In preparing raw applesauce, the amount of lemon juice to add depends on the tartness of the apples you are using. Taste the mixture before adding the lemon juice.

The cheese at lunch is, of course, for protein. Swiss cheese is made from partly skimmed milk.

Breakfast

    raw applesauce (place 1 apple per person, cored, unpeeled
        and chopped, in blender with lemon juice, honey or brown
        sugar to taste; blend and chill)
    skim milk cottage cheese

whole wheat toast with *cinnamon sugar
beverage

Lunch

*chicken soup with rice
slice of Swiss cheese
raw sliced cauliflower
Italian bread or breadsticks
whole orange
beverage

Supper

beef consommé
*braised lamb shanks
new potatoes (steamed, rolled in small amount of margarine, chopped parsley, salt and pepper)
salad: raw spinach, red onion rings, Boston lettuce, lemon
juice
mandarin orange sections, grapes and honey are dessert.
beverage

PLAN #9

Cooked whole grain cereal should be a standard item on your
breakfast list. It's a good source of many nutrients hard to come
by in the rest of our diet. It's also a good source of fiber. Vary
it with nuts, raisins, cinnamon, brown sugar, and other additions.

Breakfast

whole orange
cooked oatmeal with nuts and raisins
beverage

Lunch

beef bouillon with chopped scallions and celery
roast beef on rye bread with raw spinach
whole-berry cranberry sauce
beverage

Supper

  tomato juice
  *baked flounder with onions
  rutabaga (peeled, cubed, steamed and mashed with salt and
    pepper, bit of brown sugar, cinnamon)
  sliced green pepper with chopped scallions and fresh lime
    juice
  applesauce with chopped walnuts
  beverage

PLAN #10

Most pot roasts call for potatoes, onions and carrots, or sometimes green beans and mushrooms. Try substituting one of the
cruciferous vegetables for the potatoes or green beans. Experiment
with your own combinations. If you don't want the stronger flavors
of broccoli or cauliflower to permeate the other vegetables, steam
the broccoli or cauliflower separately and add them at the last
minute. Or serve them separately, spooning the sauce from the pot
roast over them to see if you like the blend of flavors. If you do,
serve all the vegetables together next time you make this dish.

Breakfast

  whole orange
  cooked cream of wheat with raisins and brown sugar
  oatmeal toast
  beverage

Lunch

  tuna salad with thinly sliced cucumber and lettuce on rye
    bread (tuna mixed with skim milk yogurt, finely chopped
    celery and scallion)
  whole banana
  beverage

Supper

  vegetable juice
  pot roast with vegetables (onions, tomatoes, carrots, green

beans, potatoes, celery, as preferred; cauliflower or broccoli precooked and added at last minute)
sliced green pepper and lettuce
*plum cake
beverage

PLAN #11

It's fun to have steak for breakfast on a special occasion.
Choose a very lean piece of meat and carefully trim before cooking. It should, of course, be your only red meat for the day.

Breakfast

tomato juice
small, lean beefsteak, broiled
hash brown potatoes (cook sliced onion and potato in small
amount of oil, covered; when almost done, remove cover
to brown, add salt and pepper)
beverage

Lunch

green grapes
*nut butter and sliced raw apple rings on whole wheat bread
celery sticks
beverage

Supper

beef bouillon with finely chopped celery
*marinated halibut steaks
steamed broccoli with lemon juice
salad: romaine, chopped raw scallions and celery, sliced
cooked beets, sliced raw mushrooms with lemon juice
frozen raspberries on plain *angelfood cake
beverage

PLAN #12

Spaghetti is an all-time American favorite and would be difficult to eliminate, especially in households with children. A recipe
for meat sauce is given in order to illustrate some cooking prin-

ciples that can minimize the fat content of the sauce. The truth is that the tuna sauce is a better choice. Many children also like spaghetti with plain margarine, salt and pepper; serve sliced tomatoes along with it for vitamin C. Sprinkle Parmesan cheese (which is a partially skim milk cheese) on top.

For some people garlic bread is a necessary accompaniment to a spaghetti dinner. Here, too, the fat can be minimized; buy or bake Italian bread made with liquid rather than hydrogenated oil. Use only the tiniest bit of margarine (melt and brush a mere hint over the bread). Salting the bread lightly before toasting gives the illusion of butter flavor.

Breakfast

> orange slices with powdered sugar
> oat flakes with wheat germ and honey
> beverage

Lunch

> apple juice
> sardines on cracked wheat toast (mash sardines with fork;
>   add lemon juice, salt and pepper; spread on toast and broil
>   quickly, if desired)
> cabbage-carrot salad (shredded raw cabbage, grated carrot,
>   skim milk yogurt, raisins, honey, salt and pepper)
> whole banana
> beverage

Supper

> fruit cocktail, canned or fresh
> *spaghetti with meat or tuna sauce
> salad: chicory, romaine, raw spinach, chopped green pepper
>   and herbs
> garlic bread (Italian bread slices rubbed with cut garlic,
>   brushed lightly with margarine, and toasted on rack in
>   oven)
> *strawberry yogurt whip
> beverage

PLAN #13

Turkey is a popular (and low-fat) meat. White meat contains less fat than dark meat, so it might be a good idea to use a boneless turkey roast prepared from the white breast meat only instead of a whole turkey. If you stuff your turkey, use whole grain breads and skim milk to moisten; no butter or margarine. Sauté minced onions and celery in a small amount of oil and add herbs, raisins, nuts, dried fruits, etc.

Breakfast

½ grapefruit
*French toast
skim milk cottage cheese
beverage

Lunch

mushroom-onion sandwich (sauté thinly sliced mushrooms and onions in margarine until soft; mash with fork; season to taste and spread on pumpernickel toast)
yogurt with fresh grapes
beverage

Supper

roast turkey
*candied sweet potatoes (baked sweet potatoes may be preferred)
cranberry sauce
steamed Brussels sprouts with lemon juice
celery and carrot sticks
*fresh apple dessert
beverage

PLAN #14

Get into the habit of cooking extra portions when steaming vegetables for supper. Set some aside to cool, add a marinade of lemon juice or vinegar and a little oil, salt and pepper, and refrigerate in covered jar, stirring or shaking occasionally. Drain, then serve cold as accompaniment to lunch or as ingredient in salad. Cruciferous vegetables—cauliflower, Brussels sprouts, broccoli, celery, and cabbage—can be very interesting additions to a meal when prepared in this way.

Breakfast

> gingered grapefruit (spread mixture of honey and dash of ginger or mace on surface of ½ grapefruit; bake in 450° oven 5–10 minutes)
> *walnut-cheese toast
> beverage

Lunch

> sliced turkey with green pepper rings, cold steamed Brussels sprouts (marinated in lemon juice)
> *mushroom-onion soup
> whole pear
> beverage

Supper

> consommé
> *veal stew with dumplings
> salad: raw spinach, fresh mushrooms, chopped red onions, lemon juice
> chilled pineapple chunks, sliced banana, walnuts, with sprinkle of Marsala wine
> beverage

PLAN #15

Brown rice is preferable to white rice because of its nutritional value and higher roughage content.

Breakfast

> orange juice
> cooked buckwheat cereal with chopped dates
> *bran muffin
> beverage

Lunch

> *French onion soup with French bread
> whole fresh apple
> beverage

Supper

> tomato juice
> *chicken with mushrooms and rice
> steamed broccoli with slivered almonds
> chilled grapes and pineapple chunks
> beverage

PLAN #16

This frozen dessert is for when you're in the mood to make something that's a little special. When you're not in the mood, just top yogurt with fruit or vice versa, or mix them together.

Breakfast

> whole tangerine
> *oat and wheat pancakes with fruit syrup
> beverage

Lunch

> skim milk cottage cheese mixed with cooked peas, chopped
>   scallions, salt and pepper
> cherry tomatoes
> whole wheat toast
> whole banana
> beverage

Supper

> apple juice
> *Swiss steak
> steamed cauliflower
> watercress, romaine, sliced celery and radishes with fresh
>   lime juice
> *yogurt-fruit freeze
> beverage

PLAN #17

The green beans, nuts and rice is a Cuban dish. Here again, brown rice is better than refined white rice. In addition to nutrients and fiber, it has an interesting chewy texture. For variety and to add a cruciferous vegetable to the menu, substitute raw minced cauliflower for the nuts (add at the very end of cooking so they stay crisp).

Breakfast

 cubed pineapple and mandarin orange sections
 cooked oatmeal with wheat germ
 whole grain raisin bread
 beverage

Lunch

 cottage cheese and canned apricots on lettuce
 cucumber spears
 breadsticks
 fresh grapes
 beverage

Supper

 tomato juice with chives
 *baked haddock with tomatoes
 *green beans, nuts and rice
 Boston lettuce, raw spinach and cherry tomatoes
 *spice cake
 beverage

PLAN #18

Fruit cocktail is always better fresh. Even in the middle of winter, a good mix can be made of oranges, bananas and apples with a little honey and nuts. Chilling the mixture makes it even better.

Breakfast

 grapefruit juice
 *granola with skim milk yogurt, raisins and honey
 beverage

Lunch

> tuna on hard roll (spread flaked tuna on ½ hard roll; top with
> chopped scallions and halved cherry tomatoes; add lettuce
> and raw spinach; cover with other ½ of roll)
> whole orange
> beverage

Supper

> chilled fruit cocktail, fresh or canned
> *chicken pilaf
> steamed spinach with lemon and rosemary
> *almond squares
> beverage

PLAN #19

The egg is included not to encourage you to eat more of them
but to illustrate how you can prepare eggs in a way that includes
some valuable fiber (the whole wheat milk toast).

Breakfast

> whole orange
> *poached egg on milk toast
> beverage

Lunch

> *macaroni salad on lettuce and raw spinach leaves
> green pepper strips and cucumber spears
> applesauce with cinnamon

Supper

> tomato juice with lemon wedge
> *salmon-tomato bake
> salad: romaine, chopped raw cauliflower, chopped celery,
> sliced radishes with lemon
> steamed Brussels sprouts with lemon
> fresh fruit cocktail with nuts and raisins
> beverage

PLAN #20

The "sour cream" recipe used in this breakfast is a good substitute for sour cream except in cooked dishes. You can use it in salads, dips and spreads.

Fresh fruits are ideal appetizers and desserts. If you're not used to using them for these purposes, introduce yourself to this nutritious habit by buying attractive and good-quality fruits. They can be eaten whole or sliced, chopped, crushed and blended with other fruits, nuts, and juices. Use your imagination to find variations and combinations that please you and your family. The reward is increased vitamins, added fiber, less refined sugar and fewer fats in the diet. Many people prefer fresh fruits chilled, which also helps preserve the vitamin content.

Breakfast

>   whole tangerine
>   *blender "sour cream" and honey on whole wheat raisin bread
>   (spread "sour cream" on bread and drizzle honey over
>   top)
>   beverage

Lunch

>   herring on rye toast (place drained herring on toast; cover
>   with chopped parsley and very thin slices of Bermuda
>   onion)
>   carrot sticks and raw sliced cauliflower, dipped in lemon juice
>   whole banana
>   beverage

Supper

>   tomato juice
>   broiled pork chops
>   steamed asparagus with slivered almonds and lemon juice
>   salad: romaine, raw spinach, halved cherry tomatoes, raw
>   mushrooms
>   *frozen grapefruit dessert
>   beverage

PLAN #21

An *occasional* hamburger is a harmless concession to the American way of life. Buy very lean ground beef (if you have a grinder, you'll do well to trim your own beef carefully and grind it yourself); cook slowly in a nonstick pan and serve on an English muffin made with liquid rather than hydrogenated oil.

Breakfast

> orange juice
> oat flakes with honey and skim milk
> whole wheat toast
> beverage

Lunch

> hamburger on English muffin
> green pepper and celery sticks
> sliced tomato
> whole tangerine
> beverage

Supper

> fresh grapes
> *Cornish hens in wine-tomato sauce
> steamed broccoli and cauliflower with lemon juice
> salad: lettuce, watercress, fresh parsley, chopped cucumbers
> *meringues topped with frozen raspberries
> beverage

50

Anti-Cancer Diet Recipes

ACORN SQUASH

4 servings

Cut in half and remove seeds from
 2 acorn squash
Place in shallow pan, cut side down, in
 ½ inch water
Bake 15 minutes at 350°. Remove from oven and turn squash over. In each half, place
 1 tsp. corn oil margarine
 ¼ tsp. cinnamon
 1–2 tsp. brown sugar
As margarine melts, brush mixture over all cut surfaces of squash. Return to oven, cut side up, to finish baking until squash is tender (10–15 minutes longer).

ALMOND SQUARES

16 squares

Sift together
 ½ cup sifted flour
 ½ tsp. salt

¼ tsp. baking soda
In another bowl, mix together
    ¼ cup egg substitute or 1 well-beaten egg
    1 cup brown sugar
    ½ tsp. vanilla
    ¼ tsp. almond extract
Beat well and stir into dry ingredients. Add
    ½ cup chopped almonds
Pour into 8″ x 8″ x 2″ pan, oiled or Teflon, and bake 25–30 minutes at 325° or until top has a crust. While still warm cut into 16 squares; remove from pan when cool.

ANGELFOOD CAKE

one 10-inch tube cake

Sift and then measure
    1 cup cake flour
Sift flour two more times with
    ½ cup granulated sugar
    ½ tsp. salt
Begin to beat, gently at first,
    1½ cups egg whites (10–12 egg whites)
    2 tbs. cold water
When egg whites are slightly foamy, increase speed of mixer or hand beater and add
    1½ tsp. cream of tartar
    1 tsp. vanilla
Continue beating until stiff but not dry; add, two tablespoons at a time,
    1 cup sugar
Place the flour-sugar mixture in a sifter. Sift and fold slowly into the egg whites. Pour into an unoiled 10-inch tube pan; cut through with a knife to eliminate any large air bubbles. Bake for 45 minutes at 350°. (Can be varied by addition of ½ to 1 tsp. of one or two of the following: almond extract, lemon extract, maple flavoring, cinnamon, nutmeg, allspice, mace, ginger, cloves, instant coffee, grated orange or lemon rind, or a few drops of anise flavoring or 1 cup chopped or sliced nuts.)

ARTICHOKES WITH YOGURT

Wash thoroughly
 1 medium or large artichoke per person
Slice off stem so that artichoke bottom is flat. Cut off top one-third
of artichoke. Trim with scissors, cutting off all the points of leaves
(discard small leaves around bottom). Open artichoke slightly and
place in center of each
 sprig of celery leaves
 sprig of fresh parsley
 ¼ clove of garlic
Place artichokes in deep pan just the right size to hold them side
by side. Add to the pan
 1 inch water
 1 or 2 tbs. lemon juice
Sprinkle artichokes with
 salt and pepper
Cover and steam gently about one hour, or until base is tender.
To serve, remove and discard the garlic, celery and parsley and the
spiny "choke" in the center of the artichoke. (Or you can leave the
choke in for the eater to remove when the center of the artichoke
is reached.) Serve hot with the following mixture as a dip for the
leaves:
 ½ cup skim milk yogurt
 ½ tsp. salt
 ¼ tsp. pepper
 pinch of nutmeg
 pinch of tarragon

BAKED FLOUNDER WITH ONIONS

3–4 servings

Heat together
 1½ cups skim milk
 4 tbs. corn oil margarine
Pour half of this mixture into a shallow rectangular baking dish.
Distribute in one layer in this pan
 1–1½ lbs. flounder fillets

Scatter over the fish in pan
    1 onion, very thinly sliced and separated into rings
Pour the rest of the milk mixture over onions and fish; sprinkle with
    salt and pepper, to taste
    fresh chopped parsley (optional)
Cover pan with aluminum foil or lid. Bake in 350° oven 20–30 minutes, or until fish flakes easily (onions will still be slightly crisp).

BAKED HADDOCK WITH TOMATOES

4 servings

Brush bottom of shallow baking dish with
    1 tbs. vegetable oil
Cover bottom of pan with
    1½ cups thinly sliced onions
Mix together
    1½ tsp. salt
    ¼ tsp. pepper
    ¼ tsp. nutmeg
    ¼ tsp. cayenne
Sprinkle seasoning mixture over both sides of
    1½ lbs. haddock fillets
Place fish in baking dish on top of onions. Add a layer of
    sliced tomatoes (fresh or canned)
Sprinkle over tomatoes
    2 tbs. chives
    2 tsp. dried basil
    2 tbs. vermouth or sherry (sweet or dry) mixed with ¼ cup water (optional)
Bake 30 minutes at 400°, or until fish flakes easily. If desired, after first 15 minutes, scatter over top a mixture of
    ½ cup bread crumbs
    2 tbs. melted margarine

BLENDER "SOUR CREAM"

about 1 cup

Place in blender
    1 cup skim milk cottage cheese
Add
    1 tbs. lemon juice
Start blender; add to container gradually until desired consistency
is reached
    up to 4 tbs. skim milk
Chill. If covered tightly, this spread can be kept several days in the
refrigerator.

BLUEBERRY MUFFINS

12 large muffins

Mix together
    ¼ cup egg substitute or 1 beaten egg
    ¾ cup skim milk
    2 tbs. vegetable oil
Sift together
    2 cups sifted whole wheat flour
    ¼ cup sugar
    ½ tsp. salt
    3 tsp. baking powder
Combine the beaten liquids with the dry ingredients quickly, stirring only a few strokes. Add
    1 cup fresh blueberries (or well-drained frozen or canned)
Batter should be stirred minimally, barely moistening dry ingredients, and should be lumpy when poured into oiled or Teflon
muffin cups. Bake 20–30 minutes at 400°.

BRAISED LAMB SHANKS

4 servings

Mix together in a bag
    flour
    salt and pepper
Dredge by shaking in the bag
    4 lamb shanks, trimmed of fat

Brown lamb shanks on all sides in heavy deep pot, in
    2 tbs. vegetable oil
Add to pot
    1 cup dry red wine (Burgundy or other)
    ½ cup water
    1 cup chopped celery, stalks and leaves
    ½ cup chopped carrots
    ½ cup chopped fresh parsley (or 3 tbs. dried)
    ½ cup chopped onion
    2 cloves garlic, minced
    1 tsp. Worcestershire sauce
    1 tsp. dried rosemary
Cover and simmer two hours. Add
    ½ lb. sliced fresh mushrooms
Cook ½ hour longer. Skim fat from sauce and serve with meat.

BRAN MUFFINS

about 12 muffins

Combine and stir thoroughly
    1 cup whole wheat flour
    1½ cups bran
    ½ cup raisins, nuts, or combination
    1 tsp. baking soda
Beat together
    ¼ cup egg substitute or 1 well-beaten egg
    ½ cup honey
    2 tbs. softened corn oil margarine
    ¾ cup skim milk or skim milk buttermilk
Add liquid mixture to flour mixture, stirring just until dry ingredients are moistened. Batter should be somewhat lumpy. Bake in
greased or Teflon muffin tins 20–30 minutes at 400°.

CANDIED SWEET POTATOES

4–6 servings

Melt in heavy frying pan
    3 tbs. corn oil margarine
Add and cook for 5 minutes to make a syrup
    ½ cup brown sugar

¼ cup water
Mix into syrup
    4 sweet potatoes, boiled, peeled and sliced
Cover and cook over low heat for 20–30 minutes, or until potatoes
are nicely glazed, spooning syrup over potatoes frequently. If preferred, the potatoes can be combined with syrup in baking dish and
finished in oven at 350° instead of on top of stove.

CARROT-APPLE SALAD

2–3 servings

Combine
    2 grated carrots
    1 sliced apple, cored
    2 tbs. raisins
    2 tbs. chopped walnuts
    1 stalk celery, diced
    1 tbs. mayonnaise
    ¼–½ tsp. salt
    1 tsp. sugar
    2 tbs. skim milk
Serve on
    lettuce and raw spinach leaves

CAULIFLOWER SOUP

4 servings

Place in vegetable steamer or saucepan with ½ inch of water
    ½ head of cauliflower, broken into flowerets
    1 stalk celery, sliced
    1 onion, quartered
Steam until tender. Put through food grinder or food mill. Melt in
saucepan
    1 tbs. corn oil margarine
Add and cook, stirring a minute or two
    1 tbs. flour
Slowly add, stirring constantly with wire whisk,
    1 cup heated skim milk
Add vegetable mixture and mix. Heat but do not boil. Add
    salt and pepper to taste

½ tsp. sugar
pinch of nutmeg or mace

CHICKEN-IN-A-POT

4–6 servings

Place in deep pot
   3 to 4 lb. chicken
Cover chicken with water. Add to pot
   ¼–½ cup soy sauce
   1 onion, quartered
   1 stalk celery
   salt to taste
   peppercorns
   bay leaf
Cover and simmer gently 1 hour, or until chicken is tender. Remove bones and serve meat with rice. (Stock can be strained and used for soup or sauces, or frozen for future use.)

CHICKEN PILAF

4–6 servings

In a large frying pan, melt
   3 tbs. corn oil margarine
Add and sauté quickly, stirring often (heat should be high),
   2 cups cooked chicken, skinned and cut in strips
Push chicken to side of pan, add and sauté quickly
   3 tbs. minced onion
   ½ cup coarsely chopped walnuts
   ½ tsp. thyme
   salt and pepper
Add and sauté 5 minutes
   1½ cups uncooked rice
Add
   3 cups chicken broth
   2 tomatoes, peeled and chopped (fresh or canned)
Stir, then simmer, covered, 15 minutes, until rice is cooked and liquid absorbed. If liquid is not absorbed after 10–12 minutes, remove cover to complete cooking.

CHICKEN SAUTÉ

4–6 servings

Remove skin from
    3½ to 4 lb. fryer, cut up
Shake in bag with
    salt and pepper
    flour
Brown in
    4 tbs. vegetable oil
Pour off oil remaining after browning and discard. Add to pan with chicken
    ½ cup dry white wine (or bouillon or water)
    2 shallots or scallions, chopped
    2 tbs. chopped parsley
    pinch of dried basil
    pinch of thyme
Cover pan and simmer over low heat about 30 minutes. If liquid evaporates, add water or bouillon. After first 30 minutes, add
    4-oz. can sliced mushrooms (drained) or ¼ lb. sautéed sliced
        fresh mushrooms
Remove cover from pan and cook 15 minutes longer, or until the chicken is tender and liquid is evaporated.

CHICKEN SOUP WITH RICE

4 servings

Place in deep pot
    chicken bones left from roast chicken (turkey bones also ex-
        cellent)
    2 quarts water (or part chicken bouillon if desired)
    ½ cup chopped onion
    ½ cup chopped celery, stalks and leaves
    ½ cup chopped carrot
    6 whole cloves or ½ tsp. ground cloves
    ½ cup chopped parsley (or 2 tbs. dried)
Simmer very slowly, covered, about 2 hours. Remove chicken bones (strain to remove all solids, if preferred). Let stand for a while to allow fat to rise; skim off as much fat as possible. To

stock in pot (there should be at least 4 cups; if not, add bouillon), add
>assorted one-inch vegetable pieces (green beans, carrots, celery, parsnip et cetera)

Simmer covered 20 minutes; add
>½ cup rice

Cover and simmer until rice is cooked. If available, add
>diced leftover cooked chicken or turkey

Serve hot.

CHICKEN WITH MUSHROOMS AND RICE

4 servings

Remove skin from
>8 chicken pieces

Dredge chicken by shaking in bag with
>flour mixed with ¼ cup bran
>salt and pepper
>poultry seasoning (thyme, sage, basil or prepared mixture)

Brown chicken lightly in large skillet in
>2–3 tbs. vegetable oil

Pour off excess oil and add to skillet
>1 large onion, chopped or sliced
>4-oz. can mushrooms, with liquid
>2½ cups chicken broth

Cover and simmer over low heat for 30 minutes. Add
>1 cup uncooked rice

Cover and simmer until rice is cooked.

CINNAMON SUGAR

Combine
>1 cup granulated sugar
>2 tbs. cinnamon

Store in large saltshaker and sprinkle on toast, cereal, skim milk yogurt, sliced fresh fruit, skim milk cottage cheese or ricotta, et cetera.

COD PROVENÇALE

3–4 servings

Place in large skillet with cover
    2 tbs. vegetable oil
Sauté in the oil until soft
    1 cup chopped onion
    1 clove of garlic, minced
Add and cook 2 minutes
    2 large ripe tomatoes, chopped
Stir into sauce
    1 tsp. salt
    ¼ tsp. pepper
    1 tsp. thyme
Add to pan
    1 lb. cod, fresh or frozen
Cover skillet and simmer gently until fish flakes easily with a fork.
Transfer fish to serving platter and spoon sauce over fish.

COLE SLAW

4–6 servings

Shred
    ½ head cabbage
Add to cabbage and stir well
    ⅔ cup skim milk yogurt
    1 tbs. sugar
    ½ tsp. salt
    ¼ tsp. pepper
    ¼ tsp. celery salt
Serve with
    tomato wedges

CORNED BEEF AND CABBAGE

10–12 servings

On day before serving, trim fat thoroughly and place in deep kettle
    4 to 6 lb. bottom round corned beef
Cover with
    water

Add
    6 peppercorns
Simmer gently for about 4 hours. Cool and refrigerate. When stock
is cold, remove all fat from liquid. One hour before serving, heat
    2 cups stock
    2 cups water
Add and cook until tender
    small cabbage, sliced thickly or in wedges
Taste stock; add water, stock or seasonings as desired.
Reheat meat in stock. Serve with
    prepared mustard or horseradish, as preferred

CORNISH HENS IN WINE-TOMATO SAUCE

2–4 servings

In small bowl, blend
    3 tbs. breadcrumbs
    3 tbs. corn oil margarine, creamed with wooden spoon
    ½ tsp. dried basil
    ½ tsp. garlic salt
    ¼ tsp. salt
    ⅛ tsp. pepper
Wipe and pat dry
    2 Cornish hens, each split in half and skinned
Spread the crumb mixture over the hens and place them in a
shallow baking pan, lightly oiled or Teflon. Roast for 30 minutes
uncovered at 400°. Combine in a bowl
    ½ cup dry white wine
    2 diced tomatoes, peeled (fresh or canned)
    1 medium-sized onion, finely chopped
    1 tsp. salt
    ½ tsp. sugar
    ½ tsp. dried basil
Pour tomato mixture over hens and bake 20–30 minutes longer.
Before serving, remove hens from pan and skim off fat from pan
sauce. Stir into pan
    up to ½ cup skim milk yogurt
Correct seasonings and pour sauce over hens.

DILLED BROWN MUFFINS

12 large muffins

In large bowl, combine
  1 cup whole wheat flour
  ½ cup bran
  1½ cups all-purpose flour
  1 tsp. salt
  1 tsp. baking soda
  ½ tsp. double-acting baking powder
  1 tbs. dill seed
Melt
  3 tbs. corn oil margarine
Add the margarine to dry ingredients, along with
  1½ cups buttermilk
  2 tbs. honey
Mix well. Fill lightly greased or Teflon muffin tins ¾ full. Bake at
375° for 20–25 minutes.

DINNER ROLLS

40 rolls

Place in large bowl
  1 package active dry yeast
Add to yeast
  ¼ cup warm skim milk (110°)
Let mixture stand 10 minutes. Beat into mixture
  ½ cup melted corn oil margarine
  2½ cups lukewarm water
  ½ cup sugar
  1½ tsp. salt
Add
  4 cups sifted all-purpose flour
  4 cups unsifted whole wheat flour (preferably stone ground)

  optional: add raisins, chopped nuts, sautéed onions, or wheat
    germ
Knead on lightly floured board. Form into desired shape (see below). Place in oiled or Teflon baking pan. Refrigerate 2 hours or
more. Remove from refrigerator; let rise in warm place 1½ hours.

Place in cold oven; turn heat to 400° for 15 minutes, then to 375° for 25 minutes longer. Remove from pans immediately and cool on rack, or serve hot.

SHAPES: plain—spheres size of golf ball, placed close together in large baking pan

disk shape—rolled to ⅓" thick, cut with biscuit cutter, baked on cookie sheet

cloverleaf—walnut-size balls, placed three per muffin tin

FISH AND RICE SALAD

8 servings

Combine in bowl
 3 cups cooked rice
 ½ cup finely chopped celery
 ½ cup finely chopped onion
 ½–1 cup chopped tomato
 2 tbs. chopped parsley
 1 tbs. fresh basil, chopped, or 1½ tsp. dried basil or tarragon
 1½–2 cups cooked cold fish chunks
Shake together in a covered jar
 2 tbs. vinegar
 4 tbs. liquid vegetable oil
 1 tsp. salt
 ½ tsp. pepper
 ½ tsp. French-style (Dijon) mustard
Pour oil and vinegar mixture over rice mixture and stir thoroughly. Chill, stirring occasionally. Before serving, taste to correct seasonings if necessary. Serve on lettuce and spinach leaves with tomato wedges as garnish.

FRENCH ONION SOUP WITH FRENCH BREAD

4 servings

In large saucepan, melt
 2 tbs. corn oil margarine
Sauté in the margarine for 5 minutes
 1 cup Bermuda or other onion, thinly sliced

Onions should be tender but not brown. Add
    4 cups chicken consommé or broth
    salt and pepper to taste
Simmer very gently 25–30 minutes. Fill four soup bowls ⅔ full.
Place on top of soup
    slice of toasted French bread
Sprinkle on each slice of bread
    2 tbs. Parmesan cheese
This soup is best if made the day before serving and reheated
before adding toast and cheese.

FRENCH TOAST

2 servings

Heat together until lukewarm
    1 cup skim milk
    2 tbs. brown sugar
    ¼ tsp. salt
    pinch of cinnamon
Add
    2 egg whites, slightly beaten
Into this mixture, dip
    2 slices oatmeal bread
Cook on lightly oiled or Teflon griddle until browned on both
sides. Serve with honey, maple syrup or jam.

FRESH APPLE DESSERT

2–3 servings

Mix together well
    2 grated medium-sized apples, cored but unpeeled
    ⅓ cup chopped dates
    1 tsp. lemon juice
    1 tbs. brown sugar
Chill. Serve with sprinkle of cinnamon.

FROZEN GRAPEFRUIT DESSERT

4 servings

Place together in a bowl
    1 tsp. unflavored gelatin

2 tbs. cold water
In a saucepan, combine
   ½ cup sugar
   ½ cup water
Boil for a few minutes. Add
   2 tbs. grated grapefruit rind
Remove from heat and stir the hot liquid into the gelatin. Stir until gelatin is dissolved completely. Peel and section
   1 grapefruit
Set aside 8 sections to use for garnish. Use the rest and enough more cold grapefruit to make
   1½ cups grapefruit juice
Stir cold juice into warm gelatin mixture, adding
   1 tbs. lemon juice
   pinch of salt
Strain liquid and pour into freezing tray. Freeze until almost firm but still slightly soft. Remove to bowl and beat until smooth. Return to freezer. Freeze until firm. Serve with peeled grapefruit sections and fresh mint or halved green maraschino cherries as garnish.

FROZEN LEMON DESSERT

6 servings

Boil together for 3 minutes
   1 cup sugar
   2 cups water
   grated rind of 2 lemons
Remove from heat. When cold, add
   ½ cup lemon juice
Strain. Pour into freezing tray and place in freezing compartment. When mixture is about half frozen, remove from freezer and fold into it
   2 egg whites, beaten until very stiff
Freeze again until firm but not completely hard. Can be served in empty lemon shells with mint garnish.

FRUIT AND VEGETABLE SALAD

4 servings

Slice or chop, and combine
  watercress or lettuce
  1 green pepper
  1 carrot
  1 stalk celery
  small can of mandarin oranges, drained
  small can of pineapple chunks, drained
  ½ cup chopped nuts
  salt and pepper to taste
Stir in, a little at a time, to moisten
  up to 1 cup skim milk yogurt
Serve on lettuce.

GAZPACHO

6–8 servings

Place in blender
  10–12 medium tomatoes, chopped or cut in wedges
  2 cucumbers, peeled and sliced
  3 pimientos
  4 tbs. wine vinegar
  2 cloves garlic
  1 tsp. Worcestershire sauce
  1 tsp. sugar
  3 tbs. vegetable oil
Blend at high speed until smooth. Add, a little at a time, tasting
frequently,
  juice of 2 to 4 lemons
Chill (or, if serving immediately, blend in ½ cup chipped ice).
Can be served plain or topped with chopped chives, garlic crou-
tons, diced green pepper, diced cucumbers or diced black olives.

GRANOLA

12–15 servings

Combine in large baking pan
  4 cups rolled oats
  ½ cup sunflower seeds

¼ cup powdered milk
½ cup wheat germ
1 cup chopped almonds (or other preferred nuts)
½ cup sesame seeds
Heat together and blend
½ cup vegetable oil
½ cup honey
1 tsp. cinnamon
Dribble honey-oil mixture over dry ingredients in pan; stir thoroughly. Bake at 300° for ½ hour, stirring often. Cool, then store covered. Serve with skim milk. (Can be served with honey or brown sugar, raisins, chopped apples or dates, or dried fruits.)

GREEN BEANS, NUTS AND RICE

4–6 servings

Melt in frying pan
2 tbs. corn oil margarine
Sauté until just tender
1 lb. fresh green beans, cut in 1-inch lengths (or 1 can drained)
Add to pan
1 cup chopped pecans
½ cup golden raisins
Season to taste with
salt and pepper
Spoon over
hot boiled rice

KEDGEREE (FISH AND RICE WITH CURRY)

3–4 servings

Cook
1 cup rice
in
2¼ cups water
1 tsp. salt
Add
1 lb. cooked fish (halibut, flounder, haddock, sole), broken into medium-sized chunks

2 tbs. melted corn oil margarine
½ tsp. curry powder (or more, as preferred)
salt and pepper to taste
(optional: 2 hard-cooked eggs, chopped)
Can be served hot or cold.

LEMON ICE

4 servings

In small saucepan, boil together for 5 minutes
½ cup sugar
2 cups water
Cool. Stir in
1 grated lemon rind
1 cup fresh lemon juice
Pour into freezer tray and freeze until almost firm. Use ice cold
bowl and beaters to whip quickly until fluffy. Return to freezer
until firm but not hard.

MACARONI SALAD

4 servings

Cook in salted water
¼ lb. marcaroni (preferably whole wheat)
Drain; stir in
1 tbs. corn oil margarine
1 tbs. prepared mustard
Add to macaroni, mixing well,
1 cup skim milk ricotta or cottage cheese
1 green pepper, chopped
1 stalk celery, chopped (stalk and leaves)
3 scallions, chopped (or 1 small onion)
1 pimiento, chopped
1 tbs. chopped parsley
1 tsp. basil
½ tsp. dillweed
salt and pepper
If necessary, thin with
skim milk yogurt
Serve on lettuce.

MARINATED HALIBUT STEAKS

4–6 servings

At least 2 hours before mealtime, spread in shallow baking pan
  2 lbs. halibut steaks
Mix together
  ¼ cup vegetable oil
  2 tbs. vinegar or dry white wine
  2 tbs. lemon juice
  2 tsp. Worcestershire sauce
  1 crushed bay leaf
  2 tsp. salt
  1 tsp. dried tarragon
  ¼ tsp. pepper
Pour over the fish. Cover and refrigerate, turning at least once halfway through marinating time. About 25 minutes before serving, remove from marinade and broil about 15 minutes or until fish flakes easily with fork (baste occasionally with marinade). Before serving, sprinkle with
  chopped fresh parsley

MERINGUES

about 20 small meringues

Beat until stiff and dry
  4 egg whites
Near end of beating, add, a little at a time and beating constantly,
  ¾ cup sugar
When mixture stands in stiff peaks, add, by gently cutting and folding with large spoon (*not* beating),
  1 tsp. vanilla
  4 tbs. sugar
Cover a baking sheet with brown wrapping paper. Drop spoonfuls of meringue mixture onto sheet, shaping into "nests" as individual servings (2 to 3 inches diameter) or into larger "pie" size (9 inches diameter). Size and shape can be varied to suit serving dishes, or mixture can be put through pastry tube to create fancy patterns. Bake 60 minutes at 225°. At end of baking period, heat can be increased slightly to brown meringues (watch closely). Remove from paper when cool. Serve filled with fruit, crushed, sliced or whole.

MOLDED TOMATO SALAD

4–6 servings

Stir together
    2 tbs. plain gelatin
    ¼ cup cold water
Let soak a few minutes. Meanwhile, heat together
    ¾ cup tomato juice
    1 tbs. sugar
    ½ tsp. salt
    bits of bay leaf
    dash of thyme
Add gelatin to hot mixture; stir until gelatin is dissolved. Strain.
Add to hot mixture
    1¼ cups cold tomato juice
    3 tbs. vinegar
    1 tbs. lemon juice
    ¼ tsp. freshly ground black pepper
Chill in 1-pint mold. Serve sliced with mixture of any of the following (or, if ring mold is used, place vegetables in center):
    chopped lettuce
    raw sliced mushrooms
    sliced green peppers
    chopped cucumbers
    peas
    cold cooked rice
Serve with dressing of choice.

MUSHROOM-ONION SOUP

4 servings

Melt in saucepan
    2 tbs. corn oil margarine
Sauté in the margarine
    ½ lb. sliced fresh mushrooms
    1 large onion, finely chopped
    ½ tsp. thyme
Stir into pan
    ¼ cup yellow cornmeal

Slowly add, stirring constantly
   3 cups skim milk
Cook 15–20 minutes, stirring often. Before serving, season with
   1 tsp. sugar
   salt and pepper to taste

MUSHROOM-ZUCCHINI SALAD

6–8 servings

Place in medium-sized saucepan
   4 cups zucchini squash, unpeeled and sliced, into ½-inch
      pieces
   ½ inch water
Cover and cook for 3–4 minutes, or until zucchini is just slightly
tender (not soft). Drain and refrigerate. Place in medium-sized
bowl
   2 cups sliced fresh mushrooms
Sprinkle with
   1 tbs. lemon juice
Cover and chill. Combine zucchini and mushrooms and toss with
the following mixture:
   ¼ cup vegetable oil
   1 tbs. wine vinegar
   ¼ tsp. garlic powder
   1 tsp. dried basil or 1 tbs. fresh chopped basil
   1 tsp. salt
   ½ tsp. pepper
Refrigerate until ready to serve. Stir before serving.

NUT BUTTER

Place in blender
   ½ cup nuts (pistachios, walnuts, filberts, almonds, pecans or
      pine nuts)
Blend to desired spreading consistency, adding
   up to 1 tbs. vegetable oil if necessary
   salt to taste
   (optional: add honey, curry powder, cinnamon and cloves, or
      nutmeg)
Store in jar in refrigerator.

NUT WAFFLES

4 servings

Sift together
 1¼ cups whole wheat flour
 2 tsp. baking powder
 ½ tsp. salt
Combine in another bowl
 2 egg whites or 1 beaten egg
 1 cup skim milk or skim milk buttermilk
 2 tbs. vegetable oil
 2 tbs. honey
 ½ cup chopped walnuts
 (optional: ¼ cup wheat germ)
Combine dry and liquid mixtures. Do not beat; stir just until
blended, with batter still slightly lumpy. If necessary to reach good
consistency for pouring, add
 skim milk or skim milk buttermilk as needed
Bake in preheated waffle iron until brown. Serve with margarine
and maple syrup, honey, fruit syrup or jam.

OAT AND WHEAT PANCAKES

16 small pancakes

In a large mixing bowl, combine
 1½ cups rolled oats
 ½ cup whole wheat flour
 2 tbs. wheat germ
 1 tsp. salt
 1 tbs. baking powder
Add
 ¼ cup egg substitute or 1 beaten egg
 1½ cups skim milk
 2 tbs. honey
 2 tsp. vegetable oil
Stir mixture well. Bake on oiled or Teflon hot griddle, ¼ cup per
pancake. Turn when edges look cooked. Serve with fruit syrup,
maple syrup, honey or canned fruit with juices.

OATMEAL-APPLESAUCE BREAD

1 loaf

Preheat oven to 350°. Grease and flour a 9" x 5" loaf pan (or use Teflon). In bowl, blend

     ½ cup all-purpose flour
     ½ cup whole wheat flour
     ¼ cup bran
     ½ cup packed brown sugar
     ½ tsp. salt
     1 tsp. baking soda
     1 tsp. double-acting baking powder
     1 tsp. cinnamon
     1½ cups uncooked rolled oats

Add

     1 cup applesauce
     ⅓ cup vegetable oil
     ½ cup egg substitute or 2 eggs

Mix until blended. Stir in

     1 cup dark seedless raisins
     ½ cup chopped black walnuts

Bake at 350° one hour. Turn out of pan to cool.

OATMEAL-RAISIN COOKIES

3 dozen cookies

Stir together

     1½ cups whole wheat flour
     1½ cups rolled oats
     ⅓ cup instant milk powder
     ½ tsp. salt
     1 tsp. cinnamon
     ½ tsp. mace
     1 cup raisins
     ½ cup almonds, chopped

In a small bowl, beat together thoroughly

     ½ cup egg substitute or 2 eggs
     ¼ cup vegetable oil
     ½ cup molasses

Stir liquids into dry ingredients. Drop onto unoiled cookie sheet and bake 12 minutes at 350°.

ONION-TOMATO SOUP

4 servings

Melt in saucepan
    2 tbs. corn oil margarine
Add and cook until golden
    1½ cups Spanish onion, sliced
Add to onions
    1½ cups peeled tomato, chopped (fresh or canned)
Cook tomato and onions for a few minutes. Add
    3 cups beef bouillon
    ½ tsp. dried basil
    salt and pepper to taste
Simmer at very low heat for 15 minutes. Place soup in blender and blend until smooth. Reheat. Pour into soup bowls and sprinkle with Parmesan cheese to serve.

ONIONS AND APPLES

4 servings

Melt in heavy skillet
    2 tbs. corn oil margarine
Add and sauté
    3 large onions, sliced
When onions are golden in color and slightly tender, add to pan
    3 large tart apples, cored and sliced, but not peeled
Sprinkle over onions and apples
    salt to taste
Cover. Cook 10–15 minutes. Remove cover and sprinkle on mixture
    2 tbs. brown sugar (or to taste)
Cook briefly uncovered until excess moisture evaporates. Can be run under broiler to brown top.

PAN-BROILED FILLET OF SOLE

4 servings

Wipe with paper towel
    1½ lbs. fillet of sole (or whole cleaned small brook trout or
      smelt)

Sprinkle fish with
    salt and pepper
    few drops lemon juice
Coat with
    cornmeal
Cook on both sides in
    2 tbs. corn oil margarine
Fish is done when it flakes easily. Serve with
    lemon wedges
    pan juices with chopped parsley added

PASTA WITH FRESH TOMATOES

6–8 servings

Cook in large pot of boiling salted water
    1 lb. spaghetti or other pasta (whole wheat preferred)
While spaghetti is cooking, melt in small saucepan
    3 tbs. corn oil margarine
Brown in margarine
    1 clove garlic, minced
Drain pasta; mix garlic and margarine into pasta. Dice
    6 ripe plum tomatoes
Heat briefly in pan in which garlic was browned; add to tomatoes
    2 tbs. fresh basil, chopped (or 2 tsp. dried basil)
    2 tbs. fresh parsley, chopped (or 2 tsp. dried parsley)
Tomato mixture should be just heated, not cooked. When hot,
spoon over pasta and toss, seasoning with salt and pepper to taste.
Serve with
    grated Parmesan or asiago cheese

PEPPER STEAK

8 servings

Heat in large frying pan
    3 tbs. vegetable oil
Sauté in the oil
    1 large onion, thinly sliced
    3 stalks celery, cut in 2-inch lengths
Cut into slices about 1" x ¼" x 4"
    3 lbs. steak of choice

Brown the meat in the frying pan quickly, stirring to brown all sides. Cover meat with

    2–3 cups water or beef bouillon
    ½ cup soy sauce
    1 tsp. Worcestershire sauce
    1 bay leaf, crushed
    ½ tsp. basil

Simmer very slowly for 5 minutes. Add

    2½ cups green pepper strips

Continue to simmer for 15 minutes longer. In another bowl, place

    1 tbs. cornstarch

Stirring constantly, blend in

    1 cup water

Stir the cornstarch mixture, a little at a time, into the meat and pepper mixture until desired thickness is obtained. Taste and, if necessary, add

    salt and pepper

Serve over rice.

PLUM CAKE

8 servings

Beat

    ¼ cup egg substitute or 1 egg

While beating egg, add

    ½ cup sugar

Stir in

    1 cup flour
    1 tsp. baking powder
    ½ tsp. salt

Blend together in saucepan

    3 tbs. corn oil margarine, melted
    ¼ cup skim milk
    ½ tsp. lemon juice
    1 tsp. vanilla

Add liquids to flour mixture. Stir to blend thoroughly. Pour batter into oiled or Teflon 7" x 10" baking pan. Arrange close together across the top of batter

    canned plums, halved and pitted

Sprinkle with
    ¼ cup juice from canned plums
    mixture of ¼ cup sugar and 1 tsp. cinnamon
Bake 25 minutes at 350°.

POACHED EGGS ON MILK TOAST

Poach
    1 egg per person
For each egg, combine
    ½ cup skim milk
    ½ tsp. margarine
    ½ tsp. chopped parsley
    salt and pepper to taste
Heat until steaming, but do not boil. Toast
    1 slice whole wheat bread per person
Spread each slice of toast with
    1–2 tsp. margarine
Place toast in soup bowl, top with egg, and pour milk mixture over all. Serve hot.

POACHED FISH

4 servings

Place in shallow saucepan or frying pan
    1½ lbs. fresh fish (halibut, cod or salmon)
    1 tsp. salt
    2 cups water
    ¼ cup dry white wine
    1 medium-sized onion, minced
    6 whole peppercorns
    1 bay leaf
    2 tbs. chopped fresh parsley (or 1 tbs. dried)
    1 tsp. lemon juice
    ¼ tsp. nutmeg
Simmer covered about 15 minutes, or until fish flakes easily with fork. Remove from liquid to serve.

PORK AND ZUCCHINI CASSEROLE

4 servings

Preheat oven to 350°. Grease a 10" x 6" baking dish. Brown in Teflon frying pan (or in pan brushed lightly with vegetable oil)

 1 lb. lean ground pork

 ¾ cup chopped onion

Stir in

 ¼ cup water

 10¾-oz. can condensed cream of chicken soup (undiluted)

 ¼ cup cracker meal

 ¼ cup bran

 1 tbs. chopped parsley

 1 tsp. salt

 ½ tsp. sage

 ¼ tsp. pepper

Blend well. Place in baking dish

 1 medium zucchini squash, unpeeled and sliced into ¼-inch slices

Spoon meat mixture evenly over squash. Cover meat with

 1 medium zucchini squash, sliced as first squash

Cover dish tightly with foil and bake 1 hour at 350° or until squash is fork-tender. Remove foil and sprinkle with

 4 oz. diced American cheese

Bake a few minutes longer to melt the cheese.

POT AU FEU (FRENCH BEEF AND VEGETABLE SUPPER SOUP)

6–8 servings

Place in large deep kettle

 scant 1–2 tbs. vegetable oil

Brown quickly on all sides

 4 lbs. beef with bone, trimmed of fat (brisket, rump, plate, chuck, round, shin)

Add to pot

 up to 3 quarts water

 2 tbs. salt

 2 bay leaves, crushed

 1 tsp. marjoram

½ tsp. thyme
1 tsp. peppercorns, slightly cracked
6 whole cloves
2–3 tbs. chopped parsley

Bring to boil, skimming frequently. Reduce heat and cover; simmer slowly for 3 hours. Remove meat from stock; strain stock. Return stock and meat to pot; add

½ cup chopped onion
½ cup chopped celery, stalk and leaves
½ cup chopped carrots
½ cup chopped turnip or parsnip
4 leeks, white part (optional)
4 carrots, quartered
6 cabbage wedges
4 potatoes, quartered

Simmer 45 minutes, or until vegetables are cooked. Serve the meat on platter surrounded by vegetables. Serve the broth in bowls.

POTATO SALAD

4 servings

Steam until tender
4 potatoes

Cool potatoes and slice or cube. Add to bowl with potatoes
1 onion, minced
1 tbs. chopped parsley
salt and pepper

In small saucepan, boil for 2 minutes
2 tbs. vegetable oil
½ tsp. French-style (Dijon) mustard
2 tbs. tarragon vinegar

Toss potatoes and sauce together, correct seasonings and chill until serving time. Serve cold.

RATATOUILLE

5–6 servings

Heat in large skillet
>   4 tbs. vegetable oil

Add and sauté until soft
>   2 cloves garlic, minced
>   1 large onion, thinly sliced

Add to the skillet
>   2 medium zucchini, unpeeled and sliced
>   1 small or medium-sized eggplant, peeled and cubed
>   2 green peppers, seeded and cut into strips

Cover pan and cook very slowly about 45 minutes, or just until vegetables are tender. Add to pan
>   5 ripe tomatoes, chopped (peeled, if preferred)

Simmer uncovered until mixture is thick (about 10 minutes). Add
>   salt and pepper to taste
>   1 tbs. chopped fresh basil (or 1 tsp. dried)

RHUBARB-STRAWBERRY SHERBET

8 servings

Simmer in covered saucepan until tender
>   1½ cups diced rhubarb stalks, unpeeled
>   1½ cups strawberries
>   ½ cup sugar
>   pinch of salt

Cool. Combine in another bowl
>   1 cup skim milk
>   1 tbs. lemon juice
>   ½ tsp. vanilla

Combine the two mixtures and pour into freezing trays. When almost firm, begin to beat
>   2 egg whites

When egg whites are partially beaten, gradually add, while continuing to beat
>   3 tbs. sugar

In a chilled bowl, break the frozen fruit mixture into pieces and beat until fluffy with electric mixer or egg beater; do not allow mixture to melt. Fold the egg whites into the fruit and return to freezer trays. Freeze until firm.

ROLLED OAT CEREAL WITH GRATED APPLE

2–3 servings

Place in bowl with cover
   1 cup uncooked rolled oats
   skim milk or water to cover
Cover and refrigerate overnight. The next morning, stir in
   2 tbs. honey
   2 tsp. lemon juice
   3 tbs. slivered almonds
   3 tbs. raisins
   1 whole apple, unpeeled, grated
Serve cold.

SALMON HASH

3–4 servings

Remove the skin from
   salmon (one 7-oz. can)
Add to salmon
   1 cup boiled potatoes, finely chopped
Add
   1 or 2 egg whites, or ¼ cup egg substitute
   pinch basil
   2 tbs. finely minced onion
Blend thoroughly and form into patties. Fry in heavy skillet
(Teflon or lightly oiled) until golden brown, about 5 minutes each
side.

SALMON-TOMATO BAKE

4 servings

Drain and break into pieces
   2 cups canned salmon
Break into small pieces
   4–5 slices bread, preferably cracked wheat or oatmeal
Mix bread with salmon, along with
   1 small onion, finely chopped
   1 tsp. sugar
   ½ tsp. pepper

2½ cups peeled tomatoes, chopped (canned or fresh)
1 green pepper, chopped
1½ tsp. lemon juice or ¼ cup dry white wine
Place in oiled or Teflon casserole. Top with
4 tbs. grated skim milk cheese (Parmesan or other)
Bake at 350° until bubbling and slightly browned on top. May be
run under broiler to brown.

SOYBEAN-MUSHROOM DISH

4–6 servings

Melt in large frying pan
2 tbs. corn oil margarine
Add to pan and sauté
1 small onion, finely chopped
1 clove garlic, minced
½ lb. mushrooms, thinly sliced
salt and pepper to taste
Blend together in medium-sized saucepan
1 tbs. soy sauce
1 tbs. molasses
Add
cooked soybeans (about 2 cups)
Cover and cook 10 minutes. Combine beans with mushroom mixture; heat. When ready to serve, mix in
1 tbs. fresh dill, finely chopped (or 1 tsp. dried dillweed)
Serve with plain cooked whole wheat macaroni or rice.

SPAGHETTI WITH MEAT SAUCE

6–8 servings

In a heavy deep pan, brown
2 lbs. lean ground beef
When meat is brown, pour off the fat that has accumulated in pan.
Add to meat in the pan
2 medium onions, finely chopped
2 cloves garlic, minced
2 stalks celery, chopped (stalks and leaves)

1 green pepper, finely chopped
½ lb. sliced mushrooms, fresh or canned
Cook a few minutes uncovered, then add
    1 large can tomatoes (about 3½ cups)
    1 small can tomato paste
    1 tbs. sugar
    1 tbs. oregano
    1 tsp. dried basil
    1 bay leaf, crushed
    salt and pepper to taste
Cover and simmer gently two hours. Serve with cooked spaghetti, preferably whole wheat.

SPAGHETTI WITH TUNA SAUCE

4 servings

Heat in frying pan
    2 tbs. vegetable oil
Sauté for a few minutes
    1 medium onion, finely chopped
    1 clove garlic, minced
Add
    1 large can tomatoes
Mash tomatoes slightly with fork or potato masher (or put through sieve or food mill before adding to pan). Simmer uncovered for 20–30 minutes, or until sauce is of desired consistency. Add to sauce
    1 tsp. dried basil (or 1 tbs. fresh)
    1 tsp. dried parsley (or 1 tbs. fresh)
    1 tsp. lemon juice
    ½ tsp. pepper
Add
    1 can tuna fish (7 oz.)
Flake fish with fork. If necessary, add
    salt to taste
Heat just to boiling. Serve with hot cooked spaghetti or macaroni, preferably whole wheat.

SPICE CAKE

One 7-inch tube cake

Mix together and boil for a few minutes
  1 cup water
  1 cup brown sugar, firmly packed
  1½ cups raisins
  4 tbs. corn oil margarine
  ½ tsp. cinnamon
  ½ tsp. allspice
  ½ tsp. mace
  ¼ tsp. nutmeg
  ½ tsp. salt
Cool mixture. Sift together
  2 cups sifted cake flour
  1 tsp. double-acting baking powder
  1 tsp. baking soda
Stir flour mixture slowly into spice mixture. Add
  1 cup chopped almonds or dates
Bake in oiled or Teflon 7-inch tube pan 1 hour or more at 325°.

STRAWBERRY YOGURT WHIP

4–6 servings

Prepare
  1 package strawberry gelatin
using
  1 cup boiling water
  1 cup chilled liquid from defrosted package of frozen straw-
    berries
Chill until almost set. Beat until fluffy. Fold into the gelatin
  1 cup skim milk yogurt
  drained strawberries
Garnish with
  2–3 strawberries

SWISS STEAK

6 servings

Wipe with a paper towel
    2 lbs. trimmed beef (round, rump or chuck) cut 1–1½ inches thick
Sprinkle on meat
    salt and pepper
Dredge in
    flour
Pound meat with mallet to tenderize and pound in seasonings. Brown quickly on both sides in
    2 tbs. vegetable oil
Add and sauté
    2 sliced onions
    2 sliced carrots
Add
    1 can tomatoes (about 1½ cups)
    1 tsp. basil
    1 bay leaf, crushed
    ¼ cup dry red wine
Cover and cook over low heat 1½–2 hours, until meat is tender. Just before serving, correct seasoning.

TABOULI (LEBANESE SALAD)

6 servings

In a small bowl, combine
    1 cup bulgur wheat (cracked wheat)
    boiling water to cover the wheat
Soak for about 2 hours and drain. Toss with the wheat
    ½ cup fresh parsley, chopped
    ½ cup fresh mint, chopped (or 3 tbs. dried)
    4 scallions, chopped, white and green parts (or 1 onion, chopped)
    2 tomatoes, chopped (or 10–12 cherry tomatoes, quartered)
To make dressing, combine in jar and shake well
    6 tbs. vegetable oil
    2 tbs. lemon juice
    1 tsp. salt

½ tsp. pepper
¼ tsp. garlic powder

Toss dressing with salad and chill 2 hours. Serve as filling in pita bread (Middle Eastern flat round bread): cut off 4-inch section along edge of bread in order to open a "pocket" inside bread, and fill pocket with salad. Or serve as salad on plate with Italian bread.

TUNA CASSEROLE

4–6 servings

Melt in saucepan
    2 tbs. corn oil margarine
Sauté in margarine
    1 small onion, finely chopped
    1 stalk celery, finely chopped
    1 clove garlic, minced
Add to pan, stirring
    2 tbs. whole wheat flour
Cook for a few minutes. Add, stirring constantly,
    ¾ cup skim milk
Simmer until thickened, stirring, and adding more milk if necessary. Add and mix thoroughly
    ¼ cup dry white wine
    1 cup peas, cooked
    2 cans tuna, flaked (7 oz. each)
    ½ tsp. marjoram
Mix into tuna mixture
    3 cups cooked macaroni (preferably whole wheat)
Pour into oiled or Teflon casserole. Cover and bake 30 minutes at 350°. Sprinkle over top
    4 tbs. Parmesan cheese
Brown quickly in broiler.

VEAL CUTLETS WITH MARSALA

4 servings

Wipe dry
    1½ lbs. veal cutlets, sliced thin and pounded
Dredge lightly on one side only in
    flour

Quickly sauté the floured side first in
  2 tbs. corn oil margarine
Turn and sauté the other side. Remove excess margarine from pan.
Add to pan
  4 tbs. Marsala
  1 tsp. tarragon
Turn veal once to coat with sauce. Add
  salt and pepper to taste

VEAL ROAST WITH VEGETABLES

8–10 servings

Wipe dry
  3 or 4 lb. veal rump roast, boned, rolled and tied
Sprinkle with
  salt and pepper
Dredge in
  flour
Brown quickly on all sides in
  small amount of vegetable oil
Put roast on a rack in a deep roasting pan. Add to pan
  ½ cup dry vermouth or other dry white wine
  ½ cup water
  1 small onion, minced
  1 stalk celery, minced
  1 clove garlic, minced
  1 tsp. salt
  1 tsp. rosemary
Cover; bake 2 hours at 350° or on top of stove at slow simmer.
For last ½ hour of cooking time, stir into sauce in pan
  4 small onions, halved
  6 carrots, cut in 2-inch pieces
  1 lb. green beans, cut in 1-inch lengths
Remove meat to platter. Correct seasonings if necessary. Slice
meat; serve with vegetables and pan sauce (skim off excess fat).

VEAL WITH MUSHROOMS

4–5 servings

Brush a frying pan with
 1 tbs. vegetable oil
Brown in pan
 1½ lbs. veal cutlets, sliced thin
Add
 1 clove garlic, minced
 ½ cup dry white wine
 ¼ cup water
 salt and pepper to taste
 ½ tsp. dried tarragon
Simmer gently until meat is done. Cool slightly and skim off fat.
Add to pan
 ¼ lb. sliced sautéed mushrooms
Heat and serve.

VEAL STEW WITH DUMPLINGS

6 servings

Heat in heavy kettle
 1 tbs. vegetable oil
Brown in oil
 1½ lbs.stewing veal
Add to pot
 1 cup water
 ½ cup dry white wine
 ½ bay leaf, crushed
 ½ tsp. rosemary
 1 large onion, thinly sliced
 1 carrot, sliced
 1 stalk celery, chopped (stalk and leaves)
Cover and cook over low heat 1½ hours. Remove from heat; skim
off excess fat. Return to slow simmer and add
 3 quartered carrots
 3 quartered potatoes
 2 cups peas, fresh or frozen
Cook 30 minutes longer, until vegetables are almost tender. Sift
together into a bowl

1½ cups all-purpose flour
¼ tsp. salt
1½ tsp. baking powder
Add and stir until blended
½ cup skim milk
Drop dumpling dough by spoonfuls on top of stew. Cover and cook 15 minutes.

VEGETABLE-FISH CHOWDER

8 servings

Melt in frying pan
2 tbs. corn oil margarine
Add to pan and sauté until tender
1 small onion, chopped
½ cup celery, diced
Stir in
¼ cup flour
Slowly add, stirring constantly
4 cups skim milk
Add
1½ lbs. fresh fish, skinned, boned and cut up
2 cups diced cooked potatoes
2 cups of mixed peas, carrots, corn, beans et cetera
1½ tbs. fresh chopped dillweed (or ½ tsp. dried)
1½ tsp. salt
Cook until vegetables and fish are tender. Correct seasonings and serve hot.

WALNUT BARS

about 2 dozen bars

Stir until softened
6 tbs. corn oil margarine
Add, a little at a time,
⅓ cup confectioners sugar
Beat in, one at a time
½ tsp. vanilla
1 egg white
¼ cup molasses

Sift together
    1 cup flour
    ⅛ tsp. baking soda
    ⅛ tsp. salt
Combine the two mixtures. Add
    ½ cup chopped walnuts
Bake in 9-inch square pan, oiled or Teflon, 25 minutes at 350°.
Cool slightly; cut into bars. Shake in bag with confectioners sugar.
(Variation: instead of nuts, add chopped dates, figs or prunes; add
cloves, cinnamon or allspice with dried fruits.)

WALNUT-CHEESE TOAST

4 servings

Combine and stir well
    ¼ cup chopped walnuts
    1 tsp. salt
    ½ tsp. curry powder
In shallow baking pan, uncovered, toast nuts 10 minutes at 350°.
In toaster, toast
    4 slices pumpernickel bread
Spread toast with
    1 cup skim milk cottage cheese (3–4 tbs. per slice)
Sprinkle 1 tbs. nut mixture over cottage cheese.

WHOLE WHEAT PANCAKES

2 servings

Sift together
    1 cup sifted whole wheat flour
    2 tsp. baking powder
    ½ tsp. salt
In a large bowl, combine
    2 egg whites
    1 cup skim milk
    1 tbs. vegetable oil
    1 tbs. honey
    2–3 tbs. wheat germ
    (optional: ¼ cup chopped nuts)
Stir dry ingredients into liquids. Cook on hot griddle, lightly oiled

or Teflon, until edges are cooked. Turn and finish cooking. Serve with maple syrup, honey, fruit syrup or canned fruit with syrup from can.

YOGURT-FRUIT FREEZE

4 servings

Stir together
    2 cups skim milk yogurt
    2 tbs. honey
    1 tsp. vanilla
Freeze in freezer tray until almost hard but slightly mushy. Remove to bowl; stir in
    1 cup crushed pineapple (or crushed strawberries or raspberries)
Beat thoroughly (but do not allow to melt). Return to tray and freeze until solid.

51

Favorite Recipes from the Seventh-Day Adventists

Earlier in this book there was a list giving a week's worth of typical Seventh-day Adventist meals. The Adventists, remember, are lacto-ovo-vegetarians. They eat no animal flesh, but they do eat milk, eggs, cheese and other foods of animal origin. I believe that the Adventists' greatly reduced cancer rate is due largely to their abstinence from meat, from which most of us get most of the fat in our diets.

As you know, I am not suggesting that we become a nation of lacto-ovo-vegetarians. Eating no meat is only one way to cut back on fat. Another approach—the one I've taken throughout this book—is to consume smaller amounts of fats and oils of all kinds. That way we can continue to enjoy meat (albeit in lesser amounts) and reduce our cancer risk at the same time.

However, for those of you who are interested in lacto-ovo-vegetarianism or who simply want to include an occasional meat-less meal à la the Seventh-day Adventists, I'm including the following group of recipes from an Adventist kitchen. Some of them make use of meat substitutes or analogs. Others are straight vegetarian.

Note: The Adventists as a rule do not make Anti-Cancer substitutions such as skim milk for whole milk, carob for chocolate, corn oil margarine for butter, egg substitutes for eggs, et cetera. So, though they're meatless, many of the recipes are higher in fat than they could be if these substitutions were made. Keep this in mind when using them.

BAKED OATMEAL PATTIES

6–8 servings

Sauté until translucent in small amount of oil
    1 onion, minced
Combine with
    3 eggs, well beaten
    1 can (4 oz.) mushroom stems and pieces
    2¼ cups uncooked oatmeal
    1 tsp. Vegex in ¼ cup hot water (or 1 or 2 vegetable bouillon cubes in ¼ cup hot water, or 1 tbs. soy sauce in ¼ cup hot water)
    ¼ cup condensed milk
    1 tsp. Lowry's Seasoned Salt
    ½ tsp. paprika
    ½ tsp. thyme
    ½ tsp. sage
    ½ tsp. poultry seasoning
Mix well and allow to stand for 30–45 minutes. Form into small patties and fry in small amount of hot vegetable oil until brown. Arrange in a baking dish and cover with a mixture of
    1 can cream of mushroom soup
    2 cups hot water mixed with ½ tsp. Vegex (or a vegetable bouillon cube, or 1 tsp. soy sauce)
Bake at 350° for 1 hour, or until done.

BAKED RICE WITH CHICKEN ANALOG

6–8 servings

Sauté in small amount of oil until lightly browned
    1 cup diced celery
    ½ cup diced onion
Add and sauté 1 or 2 minutes longer
    1 can (4 oz.) mushroom stems and pieces
Combine and mix well with

2 cups cooked brown rice
1 can cream of mushroom soup
½ tsp. salt
⅓ cup milk
1 can (13 oz.) Worthington Soyameat Chicken Style (or 2
 cups frozen chicken-style soya, diced)
Pour into well-greased (or nonstick) baking dish. Sprinkle with
bread crumbs. Bake at 350° for 45 minutes, or until done.

BAKED TAMALE

6 servings

Sauté in small amount of oil
 1 large onion, chopped
 1 green pepper, chopped
 3 cloves garlic, minced
Combine and mix well with
 3 cups canned tomatoes
 2 cups canned or frozen corn
 ¼ cup chopped olives
 ½ tsp. cumin
 ¼ tsp. cayenne
 ¾ cup cornmeal
 ¾ tsp. salt
 3 eggs, beaten
Pour into well-greased (or nonstick) baking dish. Bake at 350°
for 45 minutes, or until done.

CARROT ROAST

6 servings

Combine
 ½–¾ cup peanut butter
 1 cup milk (or 1 cup tomato juice)
Sauté in small amount of oil
 1 small onion, diced
 2 tbs. parsley, chopped
Combine first four ingredients and mix well with
 1 cup grated raw carrots
 1 cup cooked brown rice

2 eggs, beaten until frothy
½ tsp. sage (or more if you like a sagey flavor)
¾ tsp. salt
½ cup whole wheat bread crumbs
Pour into lightly greased (or nonstick) 4½" x 10" loaf pan. Bake at 350° for 45–50 minutes, or until firm.

CHILI BEANS WITH TEXTURED VEGETABLE PROTEIN

6 servings

Soak until soft in 1 cup of hot water (½ teaspoon salt added)
    1 cup dry textured vegetable protein
Sauté in small amount of oil
    1 large onion, diced
Add to the onion
    1 tsp. chili powder
Combine with drained textured vegetable protein and sauté another 5 minutes. Add
    1 can (28 oz.) chili beans
Simmer 20 minutes, or until flavors are blended.

COTTAGE CHEESE LOAF

10 servings

In a large skillet, melt
    1 stick (½ cup) corn oil margarine
Sauté in the margarine
    1 large onion, chopped
Combine with
    3 packages George Washington Broth Seasoning (substitute McKay's Beef Seasoning or imitation bouillon)
    5 eggs, well beaten
    4 cups cottage cheese
    1 cup chopped walnuts
    4 cups Special K cereal
Pour into lightly greased (or nonstick) 2-quart casserole. Bake at 350° for 1 hour.

DINNER ROUNDS

4–6 servings

Dip into breading meal or brewer's yeast flakes contents of
    1 large can (15 oz.) textured vegetable protein dinner rounds
    (or Worthington Choplets, Battle Creek Steaks, or sliced
    home-made gluten)
Fry in small amount of oil until golden brown. Then arrange in
lightly greased (or nonstick) casserole. Cover with
    1 can mushroom soup diluted with 1 cup milk
Bake in 375° oven for 30–40 minutes.

FAVORITE NOODLES

6–8 servings

Sauté for 4 to 6 minutes in small amount of oil
    1 can (4 oz.) mushroom stems and pieces
    1½ cups celery, diced
    1 pound frozen Worthington Chicken (analog), diced
Do not overcook. Add
    1 can mushroom soup
    5 oz. frozen peas, uncooked
    2 tbs. corn oil margarine
    ½ tsp. McKay's Chicken Seasoning
    Salt to taste
Heat until bubbly. While mixture is heating, cook as directed on
package
    8 oz. noodles
Drain noodles. Combine with chicken analog mixture. Stir to mix
well and serve.

GLUTEN

16–20 servings

(Gluten is wheat protein.)
Mix with 3½ cups cold water and knead well as for bread until
stiff
    8 cups wheat flour (high gluten content or hard wheat flour)
Form into a ball, cover with water and let stand for two hours or

overnight in the refrigerator. This sets the gluten and loosens the starch. Wash out the starch by kneading the dough under fresh running water. (Another way to wash out the starch is to put the dough in a flour sack, tie shut, and place in a washing machine that has been thoroughly rinsed first. Run the machine through a wash cycle until the water runs clear and the dough feels firm and rubbery.)

Place gluten on board to drain. Form into a "log" and cut with a sharp knife into ½-inch slices. Cook in either of the following broths.

Broth # 1 for Dark Gluten

Combine in large kettle with tight-fitting lid
        8–9 cups water
        1 tbs. Marmite, Sovex or Vegex
        1 tbs. corn oil margarine
        2 tbs. soy sauce
        1 large onion, diced
        leaves from 3 stalks celery
        1½ tsp. salt
        1½ tsp. McKay's Beef Flavoring
        ¾ tsp. garlic powder
        1 tsp. Postum
        1 carrot, sliced
        1 potato, diced
When mixture comes to a boil, add gluten slices and cook, covered, until done, about 1 hour.

Broth #2 for Light Gluten

Combine in a large kettle with tight-fitting lid
        8 cups water
        1 tbs. vegetable oil
        1 tbs. corn oil margarine
        1 small onion, diced
        1 tbs. salt
        1½ tsp. Accent
When mixture comes to a boil, add gluten slices and cook, covered, until done, about 1 hour.

BARBECUED GLUTEN

16–20 servings

Combine in a kettle with tight-fitting lid
    1 large onion, diced
    2 carrots, sliced
    2 cloves garlic, minced
    1 cup celery, diced
    2 tsp. salt
    ¼ cup soy sauce
    1 tbs. Vegex
    1 tbs. catsup
    1 tbs. barbecue spice
    1 package George Washington Broth Seasoning
When mixture comes to a boil, add gluten slices and cook, covered, for 1 hour. Remove gluten and marinate in a mixture of
    3 tbs. soy sauce
    5 tbs. vegetable oil
    1–2 tbs. brown sugar
    1 tbs. paprika
    ½–¾ tsp. garlic powder
    ¼–½ tsp. liquid smoke flavoring (optional)
After marinating, remove sliced gluten and fry lightly in small amount of oil. Or place gluten slices on skewers, alternating with
    pineapple chunks
    pepper chunks
    mushrooms
    cherry tomatoes
    (other vegetables of your choice)
Broil until lightly browned.

KIDNEY BEAN SOUP

8 servings

Sauté for 1 minute in small amount of oil
    1 onion, diced
    ¼ tsp. minced garlic
    1 medium green pepper, diced
Combine with
    2 16-oz. cans kidney beans

1 #2½ can tomatoes
½ tsp. basil
¼ tsp. sage
1 tbs. chili powder (optional)
1 tsp. oregano
½–¾ tsp. salt

Bring to a boil and simmer 30 minutes or until flavors are well blended. Top with grated cheese. (Cornbread makes a nice accompaniment for this soup.)

LENTIL ROAST

8–10 servings

Sauté in small amount of oil
    1 medium onion, chopped
Mash and add to onion
    2 cups cooked lentils (or cooked soybeans)
Combine with
    1 cup walnuts, ground
    2 eggs, beaten
    ½ cup milk
    2½ cups corn flakes or Special K cereal
    ½ tsp. sage
    ½ tsp. poultry seasoning
    ¾ tsp. salt
    ½ cup chopped celery
    2 tbs. chopped green pepper
    1 cup whole wheat bread crumbs

Mix well. Turn into lightly greased (or nonstick) baking pan. Bake at 350° for 1 hour. Serve with a favorite gravy or sauce.

MOCK MEATBALLS

6 servings

Sauté lightly in small amount of oil
    1 medium onion, grated
    1 medium potato, grated
    1 medium carrot, grated
Soak for 15 minutes in 1 cup of hot water
    1 cup textured vegetable protein

Combine textured vegetable protein and sautéed onion, potato and
carrot with
> ¾ cup Parmesan cheese, grated
> 1 cup walnuts, ground
> 1 tbs. parsley flakes
> 1 tsp. salt
> 4 large eggs, beaten

Mix well and form into balls. Brown in small amount of oil. Then
place in a baking dish. Cover with sauce made by combining
> 1 can tomato soup
> 2 cups canned tomato sauce
> 1 cup water
> 1 onion, diced
> 1 pepper, diced
> 1 tsp. brown sugar
> 1 tsp. fresh parsley, chopped fine
> ½ tsp. chili powder
> ½ tsp. basil
> pinch of oregano
> ⅛ tsp. garlic powder
> salt to taste

Bake meatballs, covered with sauce, at 350° for 45 minutes, or
until bubbly. (This sauce is also good over spaghetti.)

52

Afterword

Throughout this book we've been concerned with diet as a means of *protecting* ourselves against cancer.

Unfortunately, and this is very important, there is no evidence that dietary manipulation can increase the *cure* rate of malignant disease. This statement is based not only on epidemiological studies; we've seen it demonstrated in the laboratory as well and in the everyday practice of medicine. Once an animal develops a malignancy, no changes in its diet will better its chances for survival. Still, books and articles reporting faddish food cures continue to be published and bought by a public made gullible by desperation.

Illegitimate information is bad enough in the way it raises hopes and then dashes them. Even more important are the problems it presents in keeping patients on established treatment routines. Too often well-meaning friends and relatives are able to convince the patient that something they've heard or read about is a far less disabling, or more natural, or better cancer cure or treatment than the one prescribed by the patient's doctor; the end result is always an unhappy one.

It has not been my purpose in this book to expose frauds in treatment. Rather, I have tried to make available some of the best and most promising information about diet and the prevention of the disease. However, I want to remind you that fraudulent cancer therapy has always been with us and probably always will be and that no matter what anyone has heard or read, the best treatment advice can come only from the medical specialist who has access to the many fine cancer research facilities throughout this country.

Bibliography

Aikawa, Kohei. "Gastric Cancer Screening in Osaka." *Preventive Medicine* 4:154–162.

Altschul, Aaron. "The Potential for a Vegetable Protein in the Prudent Diet." *Preventive Medicine* 2:378–386.

Altschule, Mark David. "Some Ambiguities Concerning Vitamins and Medical Practice." *Preventive Medicine* 3:180–184.

American Cancer Society Index of Pertinent File Material on Unproven Methods of Cancer Management. American Cancer Society, 1975.

Anderson, Dale L. "The Technology of Handling Fresh Fruits and Vegetables." *Nutritional Qualities of Fresh Fruits and Vegetables.* Mount Kisco, N.Y.: Futura Publishing Co., 1974.

Ang, Catharina Y. W., and Livingston, G. E. "Nutritive Losses in Home Storage and Preparation of Raw Fruits and Vegetables." *Nutritional Qualities of Fresh Fruits and Vegetables.* Mount Kisco, N.Y.: Futura Publishing Co., 1974.

Armstrong, Bruce, and Doll, Richard. "Environmental Factors in Cancer Incidence and Mortality in Different Countries with Special Reference to Dietary Practices." *International Journal of Cancer* 15:617–631.

Berg, John W. "Can Nutrition Explain the Pattern of International Epidemiology of Hormone-dependent Cancers?" *Cancer Research* 35, No. 11, Part 2:3345–3350.

Berlin, Nathaniel I. "Early Diagnosis of Cancer." *Preventive Medicine* 3:185–186.

Berry, G., and Rossiter, C. E. "Vinyl Chloride and Mortality." *Lancet* Vol. 2, Aug. 21, 1976, p. 416.

Blitzer, Peter, et al. "Association between Teenage Obesity and
    Cancer in 56,111 Women, All Cancers and Endometrial
    Cancer." *Preventive Medicine* 5:20–31.
Borenstein, Benjamin. "Vitamins and Amino Acids." *CRC Hand-
    book of Food Additives.* Cleveland, Ohio: CRC Press,
    1968.
Bowden, Lemuel. *Cancer of the Pancreas.* New York: American
    Cancer Society, 1972.
Bowen, R. E., et al. "Designing Formulated Foods for the Cardiac
    Concern." *Preventive Medicine* 2:366–367.
Brunning, Dennis A. "Esophageal Cancer and Hot Tea." *Lancet*
    Vol. 1, Feb. 16, 1974, p. 272.
Burch, G. E., and Ansari, Azam. "Chronic Alcoholism and Car-
    cinoma of the Pancreas." *Archives of Internal Medicine*
    122:273–275.
Ca-A, Cancer Journal for Clinicians, Vol. 26, No. 1, 1976,
    American Cancer Society.
Cancer News, Vol. 30, No. 2, Spring 1976, American Cancer So-
    ciety.
Carroll, Kenneth K. "Experimental Evidence of Dietary Factors
    and Hormone-dependent Cancers." *Cancer Research*
    35:3374–3383.
Carter, Luther J. "Controversy over New Pesticide Regulations."
    Science 186:904.
Challis, B. C., and Bartlett, C. D. "Possible Co-Carcinogenic
    Effects of Coffee Constituents." *Nature* 254:532–533.
Chan, Po-Chuen, and Cohen, Leonard A. "Dietary Fat and
    Growth Promotion of Rat Mammary Tumors." *Cancer
    Research* 35:3384–3386.
*Chemical and Biochemical Methodology for the Assessment of
    Hazards of Pesticides for Man.* Report of WHO Scientific
    Group, Technical Report Series 560, World Health Orga-
    nization, Geneva, 1975.
Chichester, D. F., and Tanner, Fred W., Jr. "Antimicrobial Food
    Additives." *CRC Handbook of Food Additives.* Cleveland,
    Ohio: CRC Press, 1968.
Christakis, George. "The Case for Balanced Moderation or How
    to Design a New American Nutritional Pattern without
    Really Trying." *Preventive Medicine* 2:329–336.

Clayson, David B. "Nutrition and Experimental Carcinogenesis: A Review." *Cancer Research* 35:3292–3300.

Code of Federal Regulations: "21 Food and Drugs," Part 10–199, revised as of April 1, 1976.

Cole, Philip. "Coffee Drinking and Cancer of Lower Urinary Tract." *Lancet* Vol. 1, June 1971, pp. 1335–1337.

Cook, Paula. "Cancer of the Esophagus in Africa." *British Journal of Cancer* 25:853–876.

Correa, Pelayo. "Comments on the Epidemiology of Large Bowel Cancer." *Cancer Research* 35:3395–3397.

"Cruciferae," *Encyclopaedia Britannica,* Vol. 6, 1962, pp. 766–767.

Day, N. E. "Some Aspects of the Epidemiology of Esophageal Cancer." *Cancer Research* 35:3304–3307.

Desai, P. B., et al. "Carcinoma of the Esophagus in India." *British Journal of Cancer* Vol. 23, April 1969, pp. 979–989.

de Waard, F. "Breast Cancer Incidence and Nutritional Status with Particular Reference to Body Weight and Height." *Cancer Research* 35:3351–3356.

Donovan, P. J., and DiPaolo, J. A. "Caffein Enhancement of Chemical Carcinogen Induced Transformation of Cultured Syrian Hamster Cells." *Cancer Research* 34.2720–2727.

Duck, B. W.; Carter, J. T.; et al. "Vinyl Chloride Mortality." *Lancet* Vol. 2, 1975, pp. 1197–1198.

Dunn, John E., Jr. "Cancer Epidemiology in Population of the United States—with Emphasis on Hawaii and California—and Japan." *Cancer Research* 35:3240–3245.

Enstrom, J. E. "Colorectal Cancer and Consumption of Beef and Fat." *British Journal of Cancer* 32:432–439.

Fassett, David W. "Nitrate and Nitrite." *Toxicants Occurring Naturally in Foods.* Second Edition. Washington, D.C.: National Academy of Sciences, 1973.

Feldman, Joseph G., et al. "A Case Control Investigation of Alcohol, Tobacco and Diet in Head and Neck Cancer." *Preventive Medicine* 4:444–463.

Finegold, Sidney M., et al. "Effect on Diet of Human Fecal Flora, Comparison of Japanese and American Diets." *American Journal of Clinical Nutrition* 27:1456–1469.

Finegold, Sidney M.; Flora, Dennis J.; Attebery, Howard R.; and

Sutter, Vera L. "Fecal Bacteriology of Colonic Polyp Patients and Control Patients." *Cancer Research* 35:3407–3417.

Flamm, W. Gary. "The Need for Quantifying Risk from Exposure to Chemical Carcinogens." *Preventive Medicine* 5:4–6.

Fraumeni, Joseph F., Jr. "Cancers of the Pancreas and Biliary Tract: Epidemiological Considerations." *Cancer Research* 35:3437–3446.

Gortner, Willis A. "Nutrition in the United States, 1900–1974." *Cancer Research* 35:3246–3253.

Graham, Saxon. "Future Inquiries into the Epidemiology of Gastric Cancer." *Cancer Research* 35:3464–3468.

———, and Schneiderman, Marvin. "Social Epidemiology and Prevention of Cancer." *Preventive Medicine* 1:371–380.

Graham, Saxon, et al. "Dietary and Purgation Factors in the Epidemiology of Gastric Cancer." *Cancer* 20:2224–2234.

Gregor, O., et al. "Gastrointestinal Cancer and Nutrition." *Gut* 10:1031–1034.

Greenwald, Peter; Korns, Robert F.; Nasca, Philip C.; and Wolfgang, Patricia E. "Cancer in United States Jews." *Cancer Research* 35:3507–3512.

Haenszel, William, and Correa, Pelayo. "Developments in the Epidemiology of Stomach Cancer over the Past Decade." *Cancer Research* 35:3452–3459.

Hakma, Matti, and Saxen, E. A. "Cereal Consumption in Gastric Cancer." *International Journal of Cancer* 2:265–268.

Hankin, Jean H.; Nomura, Abraham; and Rhoads, George G. "Dietary Patterns among Men of Japanese Ancestry in Hawaii." *Cancer Research* 35:3259–3264.

Hayes, K. C., and Hegsted, D. Mark. "Toxicity of the Vitamins." *Toxicants Occurring Naturally in Foods.* Second Edition. Washington, D.C.: National Academy of Sciences, 1973.

Hegsted, D. Mark. "Relevance of Animal Studies to Human Disease." *Cancer Research* 35:3537–3539.

Heinze, P. H. "The Influence of Storage, Transportation, and Marketing Conditions on Composition and Nutritional Value of Fruits and Vegetables." *Nutritional Qualities of Fresh Fruits and Vegetables.* Mount Kisco, N.Y.: Futura Publishing Co., 1974.

Hennekens, C. H., et al. "Coffee Drinking and Death Due to Coronary Heart Disease." *New England Journal of Medicine* 294:633–636.

Hill, Michael J. "Metabolic Epidemiology of Dietary Factors in Large Bowel Cancer." *Cancer Research* 35:3398–3402.

————. "Steroid Nuclear Dehydrogenation and Colon Cancer." *American Journal of Clinical Nutrition* 27:1475–1480.

————, et al. "Bacteria and the Etiology of Cancer of the Large Bowel." *Lancet* Vol. 1, Jan. 1971, pp. 95–100.

————. "Bile Acids and Clostridia in Patient with Cancer of the Large Bowel." *Lancet* Vol. 1, Mar. 8, 1975, pp. 535–542.

Hirayama, Takeshi. "Epidemiology of Cancer of the Stomach with Special Reference to Its Recent Decrease in Japan." *Cancer Research* 35:3450–3463.

Hoover, Robert, et al. "Menopausal Estrogens and Birth Cancer." *New England Journal of Medicine* 295:11–17.

Hoover, Sam R. "Research into Food from Animal Sources—One Control Level and Type of Fat." *Preventive Medicine* 2:346–360.

————. "Research into Food from Animal Sources—Two Recent Developments in the Beef and Dairy Products." *Preventive Medicine* 2:361–365.

Hopper, Paul F. "Food Industry's View of the Regulatory Climate for Prudent Diet Foods." *Preventive Medicine* 2:397–402.

Hormozdiari, H.; Day, N. E.; Aramesh, B.; and Mahboubi, E. "Dietary Factors and Esophageal Cancer in the Caspian Littoral of Iran." *Cancer Research* 35:3493–3498.

Howell, Margaret A. "Diet as an Etiological Factor in the Development of Cancers of the Colon and Rectum." *Journal of Chronic Diseases* 28:67–80.

————. "Factor Analysis of International Cancer Mortality Data and Per Capita Food Consumption." *British Journal of Cancer* 29:328–336.

Irving, Doreen, and Brasar, B. S. "Fibre and Cancer of the Colon." *British Journal of Cancer* 28:31–32.

Jensen, Elwood V. "Estrogen Receptors in Hormone-dependent Breast Cancers." *Cancer Research* 35:3362–3364.

Jick, H., et al. "Coffee and Myocardial Infarction." *New England Journal of Medicine* 289:63–67.

Johnson, Ogden C. "Present and Proposed Regulations Affecting Marketing of Prudent Diet Foods." *Preventive Medicine* 2:403–406.

Jukes, Thomas H. "Cyclamate Sweeteners." *Journal of the American Medical Association* 236:1987–1989.

———. "Pros and Cons in the Case for DDT." *Preventive Medicine* 1:400–408.

———. "Diethylstilbestrol in Beef Production: What Is the Risk to Consumers?" *Preventive Medicine* 5:438–452.

Kessler, Irving I. "Cancer Mortality among Diabetics." *Journal of the National Cancer Institute* 44:673–698.

King, C. G., and Burns, J. J., Editors. *Second Conference on Vitamin C.* Annals of New York Academy of Sciences, Vol. 258, 1975.

Kirby, K. S. "Induction of Tumours by Tannin Extracts." *British Journal of Cancer* 14:147–150.

Krain, Lawrence S. "The Rising Incidence of Cancer of the Pancreas from Epidemiological Studies." *Journal of Chronic Diseases* 23:685–690.

Krasner, N., and Dymock, I. W. "Ascorbic Acid Deficiency in Malignant Diseases, A Clinical and Biochemical Study," *British Journal of Cancer* 30:142–150.

Krause, Marie V., and Hunscher, Martha A. *Food Nutrition and Diet Therapy.* Toronto: W. B. Saunders Co., 1972.

Krayball, H. F., and Shimkin, M. D. "Carcinogenesis Related to Foods Contaminated by Processing and Fungal Metabolites." *Advances in Cancer Research* 8:194–215.

Kurihara, Minoru. "Tea Gruel as a Possible Factor in Cancer of the Esophagus." *Indian Journal of Cancer* 11:232–233.

Larsson, Lars-Gunnar; Sandstrom, Anita; and Westling, Per. "Relationship of Plummer-Vinson's Disease to Cancer of the Upper Alimentary Tract in Sweden." *Cancer Research* 35:3308–3316.

Lasnitzki, Ilse, and Goodman, DeWitt S. "Inhibition of the Effects of Methylcholathrene on Mouse Prostate in Organ Culture by Vitamin A and Its Analogs." *Cancer Research* 34:1564–1571.

Lijinsky, W., and Shubeik, P. "Benzo(a)pyrene and Other Poly-